GERIATRIC CLINICAL PHARMACOLOGY

Geriatric Clinical Pharmacology

Editors

W. Gibson Wood, Ph.D.

*Geriatric Research, Education, and
Clinical Center
St. Louis Veterans Administration
Medical Center
and Department of Internal Medicine
St. Louis University School of Medicine
St. Louis, Missouri*

Randy Strong, Ph.D.

*Geriatric Research, Education, and
Clinical Center
St. Louis Veterans Administration
Medical Center
and Department of Internal Medicine
St. Louis University School of Medicine
St. Louis, Missouri*

Raven Press ☙ New York

Raven Press, 1185 Avenue of the Americas, New York, New York 10036

© 1987 by Raven Press Books, Ltd. All rights reserved. This book is protected by copyright. No part of it may be reproduced, stored in a retrieval system, or transmitted, in any form or by any means, electronic, mechanical, photocopying, recording, or otherwise, without the prior written permission of the publisher.

Made in the United States of America

Library of Congress Cataloging-in-Publication Data

Geriatric clinical pharmacology.

   Based in part on a symposium entitled
"Pharmacology and the aging individual" held in
St. Louis, Mo., Sept. 1985.
   Includes index.
   1. Geriatric pharmacology—Congresses.
2. Hypertension—Age factors—Congresses.
3. Senile dementia—Chemotherapy—Congresses.
4. Communicable diseases—Age factors—Congresses.
I. Wood, W. Gibson, 1945-   II. Strong, Randy.
[DNLM: 1. Aging—drug effects. 2. Drug Therapy—
in old age. 3. Pharmacology, Clinical—in old age.
WT 100 G36613]
RC953.7.G46   1987   615.5'8'0880565   86-28036
ISBN 0-88167-252-1

   The material contained in this volume was submitted as previously unpublished material, except in the instances in which credit has been given to the source from which some of the illustrative material was derived.
   Papers or parts thereof have been used as camera-ready copy as submitted by the authors whenever possible; when retyped, they have been edited by the editorial staff only to the extent considered necessary for the assistance of an international readership. The views expressed and the general style adopted remain, however, the responsibility of the named authors. Great care has been taken to maintain the accuracy of the information contained in this volume. However, neither Raven Press nor the editors can be held responsible for errors or for any consequences arising from the use of information contained herein.
   Materials appearing in this book prepared by individuals as part of their official duties as U.S. Government employees are not covered by the above-mentioned copyright.
   Authors were themselves responsible for obtaining the necessary permission to reproduce copyright material from other sources.

Preface

It is now well recognized that the aged, those 65 years of age or older, are increasing in number relative to other age groups in the population. This phenomenon has become a matter of concern to health care providers because, on a per capita basis, the aged appear in outpatient facilities 50% more often than younger age groups, stay three times as long in acute-care inpatient hospitals, and occupy more than 90% of the long-term-care beds in the United States. Also, although the aged represent at present only 10% of the population, they receive 25% of all prescribed drugs. The increased use of medications in the elderly is a matter for concern to health care professionals and scientists. The pattern of biological changes that takes place during aging may affect the pharmacokinetics and pharmacodynamics of drugs prescribed to the elderly, leading to adverse side-effects. In addition, since the elderly often present with multiple, concurrent disorders, they are more often at risk of complications from drug–drug interactions as well as interactions with alcohol and over-the-counter medications.

The editors organized this volume in order to examine pharmacological issues in the treatment of hypertension, dementia, and infectious disease, and some of the factors affecting drug response. These diseases were selected because of their high incidence in the elderly. The first section of this volume addresses issues in the treatment of hypertension. It includes chapters on drug treatment, compliance among aged hypertensives, and alcohol use and effects on blood pressure. The second section examines brain function and drug responsiveness. Included in this section are chapters on Alzheimer's disease and on the utilization of animal models for drug development, therapy, and drug-induced dementia. The third section addresses infectious disease and immune function from the standpoint of treatment of infectious disease and pneumonia, and changes in immune function that occur with increasing age. The final section discusses biological changes that occur with increased age that can affect drug responsiveness. These chapters examine drug interactions, basic studies on the hepatic drug-metabolizing system, and factors affecting adrenergic responsiveness.

This volume examines four specific topics concerning pharmacology and the elderly. Different treatment approaches and new research findings are discussed. It is hoped that this information will be a resource both in terms of clinical intervention and a stimulus for new research. Clinicians, researchers, and students in medicine, pharmacology, neurobiology, and allied health professions will find this volume useful.

W. Gibson Wood
Randy Strong

Acknowledgments

This volume is based in part on a symposium entitled "Pharmacology and the Aging Individual" held in St. Louis, Missouri, September 1985. This symposium was sponsored by the St. Louis Veterans Administration Geriatric Research, Education, and Clinical Center (through a continuing education grant from the Veterans Administration Office of Academic Affairs through the Office of Geriatrics and Extended Care), the Veterans Administration South Central Regional Medical Education Center, St. Louis College of Pharmacy, and St. Louis University School of Medicine.

We would like to thank Cheryl Mason of the St. Louis GRECC for her administrative and technical support on all phases of this project. We also would like to express our appreciation to Sandy Melliere and Yvonne Young for their diligence with respect to typing and editing, and Diane Palumbo for her creative efforts in preparation of symposium materials. A final word of thanks to the symposium participants for their contributions.

Dedication

This volume is dedicated to Cheryl Mason, Sandy Melliere, and Sharon Smith, the St. Louis Geriatric Research, Education, and Clinical Center administrative team, whose commitment and hard work have contributed significantly to the success of our center.

Foreword

On September 18, 1985, I had the privilege to be the keynote speaker for a two-day conference entitled "Pharmacology and the Aging Individual" in St. Louis, which was sponsored by the Veterans Administration, St. Louis University School of Medicine, and St. Louis College of Pharmacy. This conference brought together experts from various disciplines who are engaged in research on aging, pharmacology, and therapeutics. Many of these individuals are also actively involved in the clinical management of geriatric patients. The presentations at this conference form the basis for the chapters in this book, which provides "state of the art" reviews of important topics for the basic scientist, clinical investigator, and clinician.

Until 15 years ago, the literature on pharmacology and aging was scant and often limited to opinions unsubstantiated by clinical or experimental data. Fortunately, there is now an increasing body of research that aims to elucidate age differences in drug disposition (pharmacokinetics—the time course of drug absorption, distribution, and elimination), drug response (pharmacodynamics), and the mechanisms that may account for differences when they are observed. The chapters on liver drug metabolism during aging in the rodent and primate animal models, on age-related changes in the adenylate cyclase system, and on vascular adrenergic responsiveness in aging demonstrate that geriatric pharmacology has grown well beyond the realm of purely descriptive science.

It is important to emphasize that current research on pharmacokinetics and pharmacodynamics is limited to the study of age *differences* rather than age *changes*. The former are detected by comparisons between groups of animal or human subjects stratified according to age (cross-sectional study design), whereas the latter can only be detected by serial measurements over time in the same subjects (longitudinal study design). The interpretation of cross-sectional studies is complicated by differences in life-long exposure to environmental factors, selective mortality, and genetic variability. Longitudinal studies to determine whether aging *per se* influences drug disposition and drug response have not been performed. The studies using animals maintained in controlled environments provide support, however, for the notion that age differences may reflect what happens with aging independent of environmental effects.

Appropriately, the planning committee for the conference also sought to address important clinical problems, as well as basic research issues. These include adverse drug interactions, dementia, hypertension, and host response to infection. Chapters address selected aspects of these topics and present valuable insights for management and future research. For example, although discouraging in terms of current therapy, there has been much progress toward unraveling the mystery of

Alzheimer's disease. Surely, as more basic knowledge is acquired, new therapeutic avenues will lead to additional, carefully conducted clinical trials and, ultimately, to improved management of this devastating affliction. I was particularly intrigued by the findings that compliance with antihypertensive therapy in geriatric patients could be enhanced by the use of home blood pressure monitoring.

In response to a dramatic increase in our aged population, a demographic shift that frequently has been termed "the geriatric imperative," scientists and clinicians increasingly are interested in achieving a better understanding of the factors influencing normal aging, the pathophysiology of disease, and clinical pharmacology in the elderly. This work brings us closer to that goal. I have had the privilege of examining the authors' manuscripts in advance of publication and feel confident that they will be read with interest by those concerned with gerontology and the care of geriatric patients.

ROBERT E. VESTAL, M.D.
VA Medical Center
Boise, Idaho
and University of Washington
Seattle, Washington

Contents

Hypertension and Aging

1   Hypertension in the Elderly
William C. Cushman and Barry J. Materson

15   Compliance with Antihypertensive Therapy in Older Populations
Sidney M. Stahl

29   Alcohol Consumption, Blood Pressure, and Aging: Results from the Normative Aging Study
Robert J. Glynn, Glen R. Bouchard, and John A. Hermos

Pharmacology and the Aging Brain

47   Phenylethanolamine *N*-Methyltransferase in Normal and Alzheimer's Disease Brains
William J. Burke, Hyung D. Chung, Randy Strong, Gary L. Marshall, J. Wendell Davis, and Tong H. Joh

71   Current Progress in Treating Age-Related Memory Problems: A Perspective from Animal Preclinical and Human Clinical Research
Raymond T. Bartus, Thomas H. Crook, and Reginald L. Dean

95   Drug- and Alcohol-Induced Dementias
Gerhard Freund

Infectious Disease and Immune Function in the Aged

107   Impact of Aging on Host Response to Infectious Disease
Thomas T. Yoshikawa

115   Host Defenses and the Antibiotic Treatment of Pneumonia in the Elderly
Ian M. Smith and Todd P. Semla

131   Effect of Age on the Immunological Defense System: The Genetic Expression of Specific and Nonspecific Mediators
Arlan Richardson, Wutong Wu, Mark S. Rutherford, Dian-dong Li, Mohammad A. Pahlavani, and H. Tak Cheung

Factors Affecting Drug Response

141 Adverse Drug Interactions in the Elderly
Timothy R. McNamara

149 Vascular Adrenergic Responsiveness in Aging
Sue Piper Duckles

159 Liver Drug Metabolism During Aging: Rodent vs. Primate Models
Douglas L. Schmucker

179 Age-Related Changes in the Adenylate Cyclase System—Pharmacological and Hormonal Implications
H. James Armbrecht and Philip J. Scarpace

189 *Subject Index*

Contributors

H. James Armbrecht
*Geriatric Research, Education, and Clinical Center
Veterans Administration Medical Center
and Departments of Internal Medicine and Biochemistry
St. Louis University School of Medicine
St. Louis, Missouri 63125*

Raymond T. Bartus
*Department of CNS Research
Lederle Laboratories
Medical Research Division of American Cyanamid Company
Pearl River, New York 10965
and New York University Medical Center
New York, New York 10016*

Glen R. Bouchard
*Normative Aging Study
Veterans Administration Outpatient Clinic
17 Court Street
and Boston University School of Public Health
Boston, Massachusetts 02108*

William J. Burke
*Geriatric Research, Education, and Clinical Center
Veterans Administration Medical Center
and Department of Neurology
St. Louis University School of Medicine
St. Louis, Missouri 63125*

H. Tak Cheung
*Department of Biological Sciences
Illinois State University
Normal, Illinois 61761*

Hyung D. Chung
*Laboratory Service
Veterans Administration Medical Center
915 North Grand Boulevard
and Department of Pathology
St. Louis University School of Medicine
St. Louis, Missouri 63106*

Thomas H. Crook
*Memory Assessment Clinics, Inc.
Bethesda, Maryland 20814*

William C. Cushman
*Hypertension Clinic
Veterans Administration Medical Center
1500 East Woodrow Wilson Avenue
and Department of Medicine
University of Mississippi
Jackson, Mississippi 39216*

J. Wendell Davis
*Department of Biochemistry
St. Louis University School of Medicine
1402 South Grand Boulevard
St. Louis, Missouri 63104*

Reginald L. Dean
*Department of CNS Research
Lederle Laboratories
Medical Research Division of American Cyanamid Company
Pearl River, New York 10965*

Sue Piper Duckles
*Department of Pharmacology
California College of Medicine
University of California
Irvine, California 92717*

Gerhard Freund
Endocrinology Section
Veterans Administration Medical Center
and University of Florida College of Medicine
Gainesville, Florida 32602

Robert J. Glynn
Normative Aging Study
Veterans Administration Outpatient Clinic
17 Court Street
and Boston University School of Public Health
Boston, Massachusetts 02108

John A. Hermos
Department of Medicine and Surgery
Veterans Administration Medical Center
150 South Huntington Avenue
and Department of Medicine
Boston University School of Medicine
Boston, Massachusetts 02130

Tong H. Joh
Department of Neurobiology
Cornell University Medical College
411 East 69th Street
New York, New York 10021

Dian-Dong Li
Institute of Antibiotics
Chinese Academy of Medical Sciences
The People's Republic of China

Gary L. Marshall
Geriatric Research, Education, and Clinical Center
Veterans Administration Medical Center
St. Louis, Missouri 63125

Barry J. Materson
Medical Service
Veterans Administration Medical Center
1201 N.W. 16th Street
and Department of Medicine
University of Miami School of Medicine
Miami, Florida 33125

Timothy R. McNamara
St. Louis College of Pharmacy
Euclid Avenue and Parkview Place
and Program on Aging
The Jewish Hospital of St. Louis
St. Louis, Missouri 63110

Mohammad A. Pahlavani
Department of Biological Sciences
Illinois State University
Normal, Illinois 61761

Arlan Richardson
Department of Chemistry
Felmley Hall 305
Illinois State University
Normal, Illinois 61761

Mark S. Rutherford
Department of Veterinary Pathology
University of Illinois
Urbana, Illinois 61801

Philip J. Scarpace
Geriatric Research, Education, and Clinical Center
Veterans Administration Medical Center
Sepulveda, California 91343
and Department of Medicine
University of California School of Medicine
Los Angeles, California 90024

Douglas L. Schmucker
Cell Biology and Aging Section
and the Intestinal Immunology Research Center
Veterans Administration Medical Center
4150 Clement Street
and Department of Anatomy and the Liver Center
University of California School of Medicine
San Francisco, California 94143

Todd P. Semla
Geriatric Pharmacotherapy
American Society of Hospital Pharmacy
College of Pharmacy
University of Iowa
Iowa City, Iowa 52242

Ian M. Smith
Geriatrics Program
Department of Internal Medicine
University of Iowa Hospitals and Clinics
Iowa City, Iowa 52242

Sidney M. Stahl
Department of Sociology and
  Anthropology
Purdue University
West Lafayette, Indiana 47907

Randy Strong
Geriatric Research, Education, and
  Clinical Center
Veterans Administration Medical
  Center
and Department of Internal Medicine
St. Louis University School of Medicine
St. Louis, Missouri 63125

Wutong Wu
Department of Biochemistry
Nanjing College of Pharmacy
The People's Republic of China

Thomas T. Yoshikawa
Geriatric Research, Education, and
  Clinical Center
Veterans Administration Medical
  Center
Wilshire and Sawtelle Boulevards
and Department of Medicine
University of California School of
  Medicine
Los Angeles, California 90073

HYPERTENSION IN THE ELDERLY

William C. Cushman and Barry J. Materson*

Hypertension Clinic, Veterans Administration Medical Center and Department of Medicine, University of Mississippi, Jackson, Mississippi 39216; and *Medical Service, Veterans Administration Medical Center and Department of Medicine, University of Miami School of Medicine, Miami, Florida 33125

By the year 2030, it is estimated that approximately 50 million people will be over 65 years old (21 percent of the population) and that about 40 percent of them will be hypertensive (21). Hypertension for this group is defined as arterial pressure greater than 160 mm Hg systolic and greater than 95 mm Hg diastolic. Compared to their normotensive age matched controls, they will be at increased risk for stroke, congestive heart failure, left ventricular hypertrophy with its associated arrhythmias, renal failure, accelerated and malignant hypertension, decrease in functional IQ, reduced motor skills, and impaired activities of daily living (27,31,44). Ideally, hypertension should be detected and successfully treated when people are much younger, but this ideal has not yet been achieved.

BENEFITS OF TREATMENT

Although hypertension is a considerable factor in cardiovascular disease incidence in the elderly, it is important to examine whether treatment is effective in reducing cardiovascular complications and deaths before assuming that elderly hypertensives should receive antihypertensive medication. The landmark Veterans Administration cooperative trial demonstrated a very high incidence of cardiovascular events (63 percent) in placebo treated hypertensive men (diastolic, 90-114 mm Hg) aged 60-75 years, and a 54 percent reduction in events with active treatment (39). In hypertensives aged 60-69 years, the Hypertension Detection and Follow-up Program reported a 16.4 percent reduction in mortality and a 45.5 percent reduction in strokes with systematic and aggressive pharmacologic treatment of hypertension in special clinics (stepped-care) compared to those referred back to usual sources of care (referred-care) (12,13). In the Australian trial of mild hypertension (diastolic, 95-109 mm Hg), elderly hypertensives aged 60-69 years at entry had 39 percent fewer trial endpoints and 52 percent less cardiovascular deaths, if they were on active treatment instead of placebo (35). The recently completed European Working Party on High Blood Pressure in the Elderly Trial reported a 38 percent reduction in cardiovascular deaths, a 43 percent reduction in cerebrovascular deaths (not statistically significant), and 47 percent reduction in cardiac mortality that included a 60 percent reduction in deaths from myocardial infarction (2). In the recently reported Medical Research Council's (United Kingdom) trial in mild hypertension (diastolic, 90-109 mm Hg), the age group studied was relatively young (35-64 years) and the data have not been analyzed according to age (25). However, the risk of developing a cardiovascular complication, including the primary endpoint, stroke, was significantly related to increasing age. Strokes and all cardiovascular events were reduced by active treatment.

It does appear, therefore, that the elderly are benefited at least as much as younger patients by the treatment of diastolic or systolic-diastolic hypertension. However, it is not known whether treatment will reduce morbidity or mortality in isolated systolic hypertension, even though those with this condition experience two to four times as many strokes as normotensives (16). To address this question, a large scale clinical trial, the Systolic Hypertension in the Elderly Program (SHEP), has been initiated in the United States and should be completed about 1990. Until then, although no firm recommendations can be made, we favor cautious treatment if the SBP remains consistently above 170 mm Hg on at least three consecutive visits.

Hypertension is only one of several risk factors for atherosclerosis. Smoking, especially cigarette smoking, is a risk factor that may equal hypertension in its vascular impact (6,25). A third major risk factor is created by the high fat and cholesterol content of the typical Western diet. Each of these three major risk factors is potentially avoidable. Intensive campaigns are needed to prevent young people from ever starting to smoke. Educational efforts are required to modify dietary intake both in terms of lipid and cholesterol content and total caloric intake. Exercise may be an important factor during youth, but even physically vigorous elderly people are unlikely to maintain the same daily caloric expenditure that they were capable of in their youth. Caloric intake, therefore, must be adjusted downward in order to prevent obesity. Important impacts on these three major risk factors are not only feasible but have actually been achieved in certain experimental settings (28). An increasingly educated North American population now smokes less, consumes fewer saturated fats, eats fewer eggs, and is more aware of the necessity for identification and control of hypertension (34). Once atherosclerosis is well-established, it may be difficult or impossible to reverse. This may account, in part, for the difficulty in most trials of demonstrating any marked decrement in the incidence of death due to coronary heart disease in middle-aged and older populations that are treated for their hypertension.

PHYSIOLOGICAL CONSIDERATIONS

Epidemiologic studies have shown that systolic blood pressure tends to increase with age as does diastolic pressure. However, in the 60's to 70's while systolic hypertension continues to increase, the prevalence of elevated diastolic pressure begins to decrease (36,37). Isolated systolic hypertension becomes more common. This increase in systolic blood pressure is not "natural". It is clearly a product of the disease process of the arterial blood pressure regulatory disorder that we can call hypertension, plus the decrease in arterial vascular compliance caused by atherosclerosis. Primitive societies that do not develop hypertension as long as they are not exposed to salt, do not show evidence of this increase in systolic blood pressure with age. If anything, in these societies there is a tendency for systolic blood pressure to decrease with age as slow deterioration of the arterial walls occurs (29). Isolated systolic hypertension is by no means benign but is rather a reflection of the loss of arterial compliance induced by atherosclerosis. This relatively noncompliant vascular system cannot effectively damp sudden changes in cardiac output or total peripheral resistance so that wide swings in arterial pressure are common in this group. In fact, "labile hypertension" is really a factor reflecting atherosclerosis and is seen far more in the elderly population than it is in the young (15). As shown by Colandrea et al. (8), the finding of isolated systolic hypertension can be quite evanescent. They found 13.9 percent of 3,245 residents of a retirement village who were past 65 years of age to have isolated systolic hypertension. When these people were re-examined, only 2.7 percent of the group had persistent isolated systolic hypertension. More of the patients with isolated systolic hypertension had manifestations of cardiovascular disease than did their normotensive cohort.

A simple formula proposed by Koch-Weser permits easy recognition of disproportionately high systolic blood pressure to any given elevated diastolic pressure (20). Systolic blood pressure should not be greater than 2 (diastolic blood pressure, 15). When systolic blood pressure is disproportionately high for a given diastolic pressure, it suggests the presence of decreased arterial compliance due to atherosclerosis.

Pseudohypertension

In instances where the brachial artery is so stiffened that pressure above and beyond the systolic arterial pressure is required to collapse it, indirect blood pressure measurement will be falsely elevated. This may result in some patients being treated for hypertension that they do not have or being overtreated to the point to where they may become symptomatic. One way to check for the possibility of pseudohypertension is to utilize Osler's test (26). With one's fingers placed on the radial artery, one pumps the sphygmomanometer cuff above the previously determined systolic pressure. A normal radial artery should collapse when the brachial artery blood flow is stopped. If the artery can still be palpated, even though it no longer has a pulse, it is markedly stiffened. In such situations, it may be a good idea to determine intra-arterial blood pressure invasively. In the long run, this may turn out to be cheaper and safer than exposing the patient to the possible risks of unnecessary or excessive treatment.

In general, hypertension in elderly patients is characterized by an increase in total peripheral resistance and a relative decrease in cardiac output. This is in contradistinction to hypertension in younger individuals where cardiac output tends to be increased and total peripheral resistance is nearly normal (1). Drug therapy should be aimed at lowering total peripheral resistance without further lowering the cardiac output, if possible. The elderly patients, as a group, tend to have low plasma renin activity (9). This may be due, in part, to decreased beta-receptor function. These patients may also have an increase in the putative natriuretic hormone thought to be a digitalis-like cardioglycoside that increases natriuresis by impairing the ability of renal tubular cells to absorb sodium. Unfortunately, this natriuretic hormone renders resistance, arteriolar smooth muscle cells more leaky to sodium, impairs their efficiency in pumping calcium out of the cell, increases intracellular calcium concentration, makes cellular tone and contractility higher and, thereby, increases total peripheral resistance. This defect may be one of the causes of essential hypertension (5). Patients with low plasma renin activity characteristically respond well to diuretic drugs and less well to drugs such as beta-adrenergic blocking agents or converting enzyme inhibitors (4,10,43). Older patients have higher circulating levels of catecholamines which are capable of binding to beta-receptors (30). For reasons still not completely clear, beta-responsivity is less than in younger patients with the same number of membrane receptors. Baroreflex function, especially with respect to heart rate response, is also decreased in the elderly (24).

Secondary Hypertension

Just as with younger patients, the vast majority of elderly hypertensives have primary or essential hypertension. One can expect to find more hypertension due to chronic renal disease, but this is readily diagnosed. Elderly patients are certainly more susceptible to renal artery stenosis due to atherosclerosis. This should be suspected in elderly patients who have a sudden new onset of hypertension, sudden exacerbation of relatively easily controlled hypertension, or those who present with severe accelerated or malignant hypertension. Finding an abdominal bruit is of some value especially if it has both systolic and diastolic components, radiates to one side, or can be heard in the costovertebral angle. Renal artery stenosis is now a treatable disease even in patients with some degree of renal failure and its diagnosis should be pursued vigorously (32,38). Renal arteriograms should be performed by a skilled interventive radiologist who is prepared to do percutaneous transluminal angioplasty. Some of these lesions recur after this procedure, but can be repeated, if necessary.

Although pheochromocytoma is rare, it can occur in elderly patients, and may be more easily missed. A useful screening test is the 24-hour collection (or even a spot collection) of urine for metanephrine to creatinine ratio (17). If the ratio is greater than one, pheochromocytoma should be suspected. Computerized tomography remains the best noninterventive definitive test for localizing a pheochromocytoma.

Elderly patients are more likely to have diastolic hypertension due to marked hypothyroidism than are younger patients. This can be a particularly devastating disease because the combination of hypertension with hyperlipidemia characteristic of myxedema is markedly vasculotoxic. Such patients may experience disabling angina pectoris or even myocardial infarction when their metabolic rate is returned toward normal by administration of thyroid hormone.

Sudden unexplained increases in blood pressure associated with equally inexplicable decreases in renal function may be clues to cholesterol embolization into the kidneys (19). Such patients generally have diffuse atherosclerotic disease and may have abdominal aortic aneurysms. They may or may not have symptoms of cholesterol embolization to other peripheral vascular beds such as the lower extremities (patchy dry gangrene), the brain (transient ischemic attacks) or the eye (amaurosis fugax). Hypertension resulting from renal cholesterol embolization must be carefully controlled. If an abdominal aortic aneurysm is identified by ultrasound and is large and the patient is a surgical candidate, prevention of further embolization requires removal of the aneurysm. Renal biopsy may be considered in such patients if the pathologist is instructed to seek cholesterol emboli carefully. Old age alone is not a contraindication to renal biopsy (33).

SPECIAL CONSIDERATIONS FOR THERAPY

Just as physicians must make modifications of drug dose and administration for the pediatric population, so must they for the geriatric population.

Compliance

When a patient is seen by several different physicians, as is frequently the case in the geriatric population, there is an opportunity for prescription of a multiplicity of drugs that may be difficult and confusing to take and sometimes with counteracting beneficial effects or additive adverse effects. The physician treating geriatric hypertensive patients has a special obligation to compile and maintain a current list of all medications that a patient is taking including those purchased without a prescription. Either the patient or a family member who participates in their health care should be asked to bring all medications that the patient is taking on every visit. A few minutes spent reviewing each of the medications is frequently rewarded by the discovery that the medication is not being taken as prescribed. Medications that are no longer necessary, are hazardous, or that are actively interfering with the treatment of the patient should be discarded in the office with the permission of the patient. Every effort should be made to provide medications either once daily or not more than twice daily. Specific routine should be set up for medication dosing. If the patient is not fully oriented, assistance of a competent family member or visiting nurse should be enlisted. Sometimes, a greater risk than noncompliance is over-compliance due to patients forgetting that they have already taken their medication dose and repeating that dose. Patients should be specifically told that they may not give their medications to anyone else nor may they accept medication of any kind from another individual. Let them know that you will be happy to discuss any medication with them and that they should call you for a presumed side effect rather than stopping the medication until their next office visit.

Geriatric patients may be particularly sensitive to medications such as diuretics. The lowest available dose should be used initially and then titrated upward only as needed. Geriatric patients frequently have concomitant diseases with their hypertension. Whenever possible, an antihypertensive agent that is also effective for the concomitant disease should be selected. One example would be the use of a nonselective beta-adrenergic blocking agent for the patient with hypertension and essential familial tremor.

There is a small group of geriatric hypertensive patients who do not have pseudohypertension but who are exceedingly brittle in their response to treatment. These patients are characterized by having marked swings in response to an increase or a decrease in antihypertensive drug dose. They also tend to have particularly wide blood pressure swings in response to stress. Considerable experience with these patients has allowed us to elaborate several useful guidelines. Do not insist upon absolute perfection in blood pressure control. You probably cannot achieve it and will only harm the patient by attempting to do so. Do not over react. These patients characteristically become upset by events at home with children, grandchildren, neighbors, etc. If they come to the office excited or upset, and their blood pressure is higher than usual, we generally do not increase the drugs. It is imperative to determine standing blood pressure in these patients. Such patients tend to be quite intolerant to orthostatic falls in blood pressure and it may well be necessary to accept higher supine blood pressures in order to have acceptable standing pressures. By and large, these patients are in their eighth and ninth decade of life and have defined themselves as survivors. Treatment of blood pressure and the expectation of doing good cannot be permitted to impinge upon what is frequently an already limited life style.

Urinary outflow obstruction is a frequently overlooked problem in geriatric patients. Increased sympathetic nervous system discharge may occur when the urinary bladder contains more than 300 ml of urine. It is sometimes possible to normalize or reduce hypertension simply by draining the bladder or by providing operative relief of outlet obstruction. Careful palpation of the suprapubic area should be part of the physical examination of hypertensive geriatric patients.

There are many other pharmacologic considerations that are relevant to treatment of hypertension in the geriatric patient. Standard doses of drugs for younger patients may either be over-effective or under-effective in the elderly. Ordinarily, potent loop-blocking diuretics should not be used in the elderly because of the risk of excessive volume depletion, orthostatic hypotension, and symptomatic hypokalemia. Levels of serum albumin may be lower and there may be considerable competition for binding sites by other drugs. Therefore, it is possible for drugs to have higher free plasma levels and thus exert more of an effect than anticipated.

Potassium metabolism is of considerable importance in the geriatric patient. Older patients who have some decrement in glomerular filtration rate and who usually have diabetes mellitus may also have type IV renal tubular acidosis (hyporeninemic hypoaldosteronism). These patients frequently have high normal to above normal serum potassium levels and may be at serious risk for hyperkalemia if they are treated with potassium-sparing diuretic drugs or potassium supplements. Patients with organic heart disease who become hypokalemic may be at risk for a greater frequency and severity of ventricular ectopic activity (7).

The reduced baroreceptor activity in geriatric patients predisposes them to postural hypotension. However, one advantage of this change is that, unlike younger patients, they may have less or no tachycardia in response to direct vasodilator drugs such as hydralazine. This provides an advantage of being able to treat such patients with a diuretic plus a direct vasodilating agent without the necessity for a concomitant beta-adrenergic blocking agent.

Geriatric patients may have subtle left ventricular dysfunction that may be exacerbated by drugs with a negative inotropic or chronotropic effect such as beta-adrenergic blocking agents or verapamil. In addition, those patients with pre-existing left ventricular hypertrophy are more susceptible to ventricular dysrhythmias associated with hypokalemia.

Elderly patients are more likely to have peripheral arterial disease with symptomatic intermittent claudication. Some of these patients may have an increase in their symptoms associated with antihypertensive drugs that decrease cardiac output. The beta-adrenergic blocking agents in particular, may be associated with cold extremities and even Raynaud's phenomenon.

Concomitant organ system dysfunction is likely to be more common in this population. In addition to the risk of subtle or even overt dementia and its consequences for compliance, one must consider susceptibility to confusion or depression associated with drugs that have their primary effect in the central nervous system. Blood flow to the bowel may be diminished and absorption of drugs across the intestinal wall may be impaired. Hepatic blood flow and function may also be diminished. This may decrease the intensity of the first pass phenomenon for deactivation of drugs such as propranolol and, thereby, increase its potential for therapeutic efficacy. Glomerular filtration rate generally decreases as a function of age. Because serum creatinine is a reflection of lean body mass, and because lean body mass may also diminish with age, the presence of a normal serum creatinine alone cannot be equated with normal glomerular filtration rate. Drugs excreted by the kidney may accumulate and either be more effective than anticipated or have more adverse reactions. The aging kidney is less responsive to marked changes in sodium load. The elderly patient who receives an unusual sodium load by way of a salty meal or intravenous infusion of saline may have a much greater volume expansion with consequent effect on arterial pressure than a younger individual. Conversely, the elderly patient placed on severe sodium restriction takes much longer to come into balance and may become substantially volume depleted and hypotensive.

Many of the antihypertensive agents may cause sexual dysfunction, especially impotence, in a minority of patients but the elderly are especially susceptible and are often hesitant to volunteer complaints of this nature. Therefore, it is important to document a sexual history before treatment is initiated, if possible. One should then discreetly inquire about changes in sexual function after drugs are added or changed, while trying to avoid suggesting that sexual dysfunction should develop.

Treatment Approach

For mild diastolic hypertension and isolated systolic hypertension, a sustained elevation in blood pressure should be confirmed on at least three consecutive visits over a three to four month period before pharmacologic therapy is instituted (3). Some forms of nonpharmacologic therapy that may have other health benefits, such as weight reduction in the overweight or limitation of alcohol intake in those who consume more than three drink-equivalents (40 gm alcohol) daily, may be instituted before the end of the period of observation (18). However, moderate sodium restriction should be reserved for confirmed hypertension since it has no other known health benefits in nonedematous individuals. Moderate sodium restriction (4 to 6 grams of salt per day) will enhance diuretic efficacy and reduce potassium loss. Regular exercise may also be of benefit but has not been studied adequately in elderly hypertensives (18,23).

When the decision has been made to initiate drug therapy, the considerations outlined in the previous section should be kept in mind in the selection of drugs. In addition, one should consider predicted efficacy, convenience of dosing, expense, and the previous "tract record" of a drug in clinical trials and with the individual physician. Perhaps of greatest importance is a recognition of both the absolute and the relative contraindications of any antihypertensive agent that one considers initiating.

When pharmacotherapy is used in the elderly, lower doses should be initiated than in younger patients, and titration should proceed more slowly. Older patients should be monitored more carefully, especially shortly after initiating therapy, and they should seek care quickly for intercurrent illness (14).

Even though greater caution should be exercised, the overwhelming majority of patients above age 60 tolerate many antihypertensive agents well and respond well to stepped-care therapy. Virtually, all the trials demonstrating reduction in morbidity and mortality from treatment utilized diuretics with or without standard step-2 agents, such as reserpine, methyldopa or hydralazine. Diuretics are quite effective in maintaining reductions in diastolic blood pressure, but systolic blood pressure is reduced to an even greater extent, and is reduced more with diuretics than beta-blockers (11,41).

The Veterans Administration Cooperative Study Group on Antihypertensive Agents has recently completed a four-year trial of the efficacy and toleration of antihypertensive agents in the elderly (60 years of age or older) with diastolic blood pressure 95-114 mm Hg or systolic blood pressure greater than 160 mm Hg. Blood pressure was normalized with low to average doses of hydrochlorothiazide in 60 percent of patients, and 90 percent were controlled if a step-2 agent (reserpine, hydralazine, metoprolol, or methyldopa) was added for those patients who were not controlled with the diuretic alone. All regimens were generally well-tolerated. Extensive psychometric testing not only failed to show deterioration of intellect, affect, mechanical skills, and activities of daily living, but indicated an improvement.

Low dose reserpine still offers many advantages in the treatment of elderly hypertension: low cost, unsurpassed efficacy as a step-2 agent, single tablet per day dosage, continued efficacy if a dosage is omitted, and favorable side effects profile when compared to other step-2 agents (22). Hydralazine, as mentioned previously, is an excellent step-2 drug in the elderly because it lacks central nervous system side effects, is relatively inexpensive, does not produce postural hypotension, does not depress myocardial function, and is rarely accompanied by tachycardia in the older hypertensive (40,42). Beta-blockers may also be quite effective in the elderly, particularly when combined with a diuretic but contraindications should be observed carefully because of the problems mentioned previously (45).

Other agents which may be effective and well-tolerated in the elderly include the central alpha agonists, clonidine and guanabenz, and the calcium antagonists. Drugs that may be effective and well-tolerated in some elderly patients, but that we generally try to avoid because of a propensity toward postural hypotension, include guanethidine, guanadrel, prazosin, and labetalol. Methyldopa has been used quite extensively in the elderly, but it also can produce postural hypotension on occasion.

Angiotensin-converting enzyme inhibitors, such as captopril and enalapril, may be desirable agents for the elderly because of their lack of central nervous system side effects and favorable hemodynamic effects; however, they have not been studied adequately in this age group.

CONCLUSION

The hypertensive elderly are at high risk for increased cardiovascular morbidity and mortality, but there is good evidence that antihypertensive therapy is effective in lowering blood pressure and reducing cardiovascular complications. Most of the commonly used antihypertensive agents are well-tolerated by geriatric hypertensive patients, but lower initial doses and greater care must be exercised because they are at increased risk for the adverse effects that these agents produce.

REFERENCES

1. Adamopoulos, P.N., Chrysanthakopoulis, S.G., Frohlich, E.D. (1975): Am. J. Cardiol., 36:697-701.
2. Amery, A., Brixko, P., Clement, D., De Schaepdryver, A., Fagard, R., Forte, J., Henry, J.F., Leonetti, G., O'Malley, K., Strasser, T., Birkenhager, W., Bulpitt, C., Deruyttere, M., Dollery, C., Forette, F., Hamdy, R., Joossens, J.V., Lund-Johansen, P., Petrie, J., Tuomilehto, J., and Williams, B.(1985): Lancet i: 1349-1354.
3. A report of the Management Committee of the Australian Therapeutic Trial in Mild Hypertension (1985): Lancet i: 185-191.
4. Atlas, S.A., Case, D.B., Sealey, J.E., Laragh, J.H., McKinstry, D.N. (1979): Hypertension, 1(3):274-280.
5. Blaustein, M.P., and Hamlyn, J.M. (1984): Am. J. Med., 77(4A):45-59.
6. Bulpitt, C.J., Clifton, P., Dollery, C.T., Harper, G.S., Beilin, L.J., Coles, E.C., Gear, J.S.S., Johnson, B.F., and Munro-Faure, A.D. (1979): Lancet ii:134-137.
7. Caralis, P.V., Materson, B.J., and Perez-Stable, E.S. (1984): Mineral Electrolyte Metab., 10:148-154.
8. Colandrea, M.A., Friedman, G.D., Nichaman, M.Z., and Lynd, C.N. (1970): Circulation, 41:239-245.
9. Crane, M.G., and Harris, J.J. (1976): J. Lab. Clin. Med., 87:947-959.
10. Freis, E.D., Materson, B.J., Flamerbaum, W., and the Veterans Administration Cooperative Study Group on Antihypertensive Agents. (1983): Am. J. Med., 74:1029-1041.
11. Greenberg, G., Brennan, R.J., Miall, W.E. (1984): Am. J. Med., 11:45-51.
12. Hypertension Detection and Follow-up Program Cooperative Group. (1979): JAMA, 242:2572-2577.
13. Hypertension Detection and Follow-up Program Cooperative Group. (1982): JAMA, 247:633-638.
14. Jackson, G., Pierscianowski, T.A., Mahon, W., and Condon, J. (1976): Lancet ii:1317-1318.
15. Kannel, W.B., Sorlie, P., and Gordon, T. (1980): Circulation, 61:1183-1187.
16. Kannel, W.B., Wolf, P.A., McGee, D.L., Dawber, T.R., McNamara, T., and Castelli, W.P. (1981): JAMA, 245:1225-1229.

17. Kaplan, N.M., Kramer, N.J., and Holland, O.B. (1977): Arch. Intern. Med., 137:190-193.
18. Kaplan, N.M. (1985): Ann. Intern. Med., 102:359-373.
19. Kassirer, J.P. (1969): N. Engl. J. Med., 280:812-818.
20. Koch-Weser, J. (1973): Am. J. Cardiol., 32:499-510.
21. Lamy, P.P. (1980): Prescribing for the Elderly. PSG Publishing Co., Littleton, Massachusetts.
22. Luxenberg, J., and Feigenbaum, L.Z. (1983): J. Am. Geriatr. Soc., 31:556-559.
23. Martin, J.E., Dubbert, P.M., and Cushman, W.C. (1985): Circulation, 72(Suppl.):13.
24. McGarry, K., Laher, M., Fitzgerald, D., Horgan, J., O'Brien, E., and O'Malley, K. (1983): Hypertension, 5:763-766.
25. Medical Research Council Working Party. (1985): Br. Med. J., 291:97-104.
26. Messerli, F.H., Ventura, H.O., and Amodeo, C. (1985): N. Engl. J. Med., 312:1548-1551.
27. Miller, R.E., Shapiro, A.P., King, H.E., Ginchereau, E.H., and Hosutt, J.A. (1984): Hypertension, 6:202-208.
28. Multiple Risk Factor Intervention Trial Research Group. (1982): JAMA, 248:1465-1477.
29. Oliver, W.J., Cohen, E.L., and Neel. J.V. (1975): Circulation, 52:146-151.
30. Palmer, B.S., Ziegler, M.G., and Lake, C.R. (1978): J. Gerontol., 33:482-487.
31. Shurtleff, D. (1974): The Framingham Study - An Epidemiological Investigation of Cardiovascular Disease, edited by W.B. Kannel and T. Gordon, US Department of Health, Education and Welfare. Public Health Service, National Institutes of Health, DHEW Publication No. (NIH) 74-599, Washington, D.C.
32. Sos, T.A., Pickering T.G., Sniderman, K., Saddekni, S., Case, D.B., Silane, M.F., Vaughan, E.D., Jr., and Laragh, J.H. (1983): N. Engl. J. Med., 309:274-279.
33. Stemmer, C.L., Pardo, V., Materson, B.J., and Perez-Stable, E.C. (1986): Kidney Int., 29:204.
34. Stern, M.P. (1979): Ann. Intern. Med., 91:630-640.
35. The Management Committee, Australian National Blood Pressure Study. (1981): Treatment of mild hypertension in the elderly. Med. J. Aust., 2:398-402.
36. US Department of Health, Education and Welfare (November 4, 1964): Blood Pressure of Adults by Age and Sex, United States, 1960-1962. National Health Survey. National Center for Health Statistics, Series 11.
37. US Department of Health, Education and Welfare (November 5, 1964): Blood Pressure of Adults by Race and Area, United States, 1960-1962. National Health Survey. National Center for Health Statistics, Series 11.
38. Vaughan, E.D., Jr. (1985): Kidney Int., 27:811-827.

39. Veterans Administrative Cooperative Study Group on Antihypertensive Agents. (1972): Circulation, 45:991-1004.
40. Veterans Administration Cooperative Study on Antihypertensive Agents. (1981): Circulation, 64:772-779.
41. Veterans Administation Cooperative Study Group on Antihypertensive Agents. (1982): JAMA, 248:2004-2011.
42. Veterans Administration Cooperative Study Group on Antihypertensive Agents. (1983): Am. J. Cardiol., 52:1230-137.
43. Veterans Administration Cooperative Study Group on Antihypertensive Agents. (1984): Arch. Intern. Med., 144:1947-1953.
44. Wilkie, F., and Eisdorfer, C. (1971): Science, 172:959-962.
45. Wikstrand J., and Berglund G. (1982): Br. Med. J., 285:850.

COMPLIANCE WITH ANTIHYPERTENSIVE THERAPY IN OLDER POPULATIONS

Sidney M. Stahl

Department of Sociology and Anthropology,
Purdue University, West Lafayette, Indiana 47907

An estimated 11 percent of the U.S. population, or 26 million persons, are age 65 and older. This group has increased 28 percent during the last decade and will increase 36 percent by the year 2000 to an estimated 13 percent of the population. A continuing decrease in the birth rate and the coming of age of "baby boom" children account for most of this change. However, increased longevity in age categories past the fifth decade of life also impacts on both the proportion and numbers of persons over 65 in our population. While some argue that this trend will dramatically impact the disease care delivery system, others argue that chronic morbidity will be delayed and then compressed into the last few years of life (12).

The older population purchases approximately 25 percent of all prescriptions sold in the U.S. (1). The cost of medication represents the second largest out-of-pocket medical expense for this age group. The increasing role of chemicals in the lives of the elderly is strongly associated with the prevalence of hypertension in this group. While definitions of hypertension vary, an estimated 30 percent of those persons 65 and over have documented hypertension. Aggressive treatment of hypertension quickly followed results of the Veterans Administration Cooperative Study Group on Hypertension Medication which demonstrated the association between treating moderate hypertension and a reduction in morbid cardiovascular events. Of the 100 drugs most frequently ordered or provided in medical office practice in the U.S., the top 3 are prescribed for hypertension (Inderal®, Lasix®, and Dyazide®) (16).

The Harris surveys of 1973 and 1979 indicate that increasing proportions of older persons report having hypertension (21,22). In 1973, 38 percent of those persons over 65 report having been told that they have high blood pressure, while in

1979, that figure increases to 43 percent (13). In 1979, 81 percent of those who say they have high blood pressure report taking antihypertensive medication with increasing numbers (between 1973 and 1979) on salt and weight reduction programs.

While the National Health Examination Survey reports variability between self-report and actual blood pressure measurement (26), there is a clear increase in knowledge about hypertension, especially among the elderly (15). Partially responsible for these changes are the Veterans Administration Cooperative Study Group on Antihypertensive Agents and the Hypertension Detection and Follow-up Program Cooperative Group (HDFP) studies (14,31,34,35). The medical community is more vigorously treating hypertension based on reasonable evidence of effectiveness. The confluence of this aggressive treatment with increasing numbers of older people raises fascinating questions about real treatment effects. Of concern are problems aging patients on antihypertensive medication have in maintaining themselves on that therapy.

COMPLIANCE: PROVIDER, PATIENT, AND INTERACTION PROBLEM

The term "compliance" has received bad press in patient care research. The term puts all of the onus on the patient. The physician rationally prescribes a course of treatment, based on scientifically objective criteria, with which the patient is expected to comply. Successful blood pressure reduction is attributed to the physician, failure to the patient. The patient cannot win. The term "adherence" has been proposed as semantically more neutral for describing the outcome of a provider/patient interaction.

Whether we prefer "compliance" or "adherence," we are dealing with a situation fraught with the potential for error. Even given stepped-care treatment (systematic and aggressive pharmacologic treatment of hypertension in special clinics) (14,28), each patient represents a clinical experiment. The typically asymptomatic nature of hypertension exacerbates communication difficulties. Although hypertensives view their health as worse than nonhypertensives, 75 percent of the hypertensives say that the condition has no effect on their lifestyle (13). Furthermore, compliance with medical regimens is only one stage in a sequence of decisions and opportunities beginning with screening and ideally ending with long-term blood pressure control. Each stage has the potential for losing the patient to followup due to medical, patient, or provider/patient interaction errors. To ultimately achieve long-term compliance, the patient must be "found" at initial screening, allow blood pressure rechecks, seek medical help if verified, see a provider willing to prescribe, understand the nature of the problem, appropriately take prescribed medication, and continue doing so for the rest of his/her life.

Ignoring the semantics of compliance versus adherence, we also face a problem in measuring this behavior. There seem to be three behavioral categories referred to as compliance: a) reported pill taking; b) maintenance in a disease care delivery system; and c) level of blood pressure.

Reported pill taking is strongly and inversely related to diastolic blood pressure reduction (13,23,27). On the other hand, if the medical criterion is blood pressure reduction, then it seems most appropriate to use blood pressure as the compliance indicator. While some patients may be pill-compliant but remain out of control, providers usually attempt other chemical solutions to the seemingly intractable hypertension.

In our research on antihypertensive compliance, we use maintenance within the system and blood pressure reduction as outcome measures (28). Confirmed hypertension is seldom reduced without medical intervention. Therefore, a measure of compliance <u>potential</u> is the ability of the disease care delivery system to motivate the patient to return on a regular basis. Without this, we have no hope of achieving the primary objective of antihypertensive therapy. Therefore, as will be discussed later, we are concerned with techniques which first, maintain patients in the system and second, facilitate blood pressure reduction.

While blood pressure varies within and between individuals in a given age category, the VA and HDFP hypertension studies indicate the utility of treating all patients whose diastolic pressures exceed 94 (10,14,28,29,34,35). Franklin (11) cites evidence that systolic hypertension (systolic pressure in excess of 160 mm Hg and diastolic less than 90 mm Hg) produces risks as grave as combined systolic/diastolic hypertension. There is growing evidence that sustained diastolic blood pressure in excess of 90 mm Hg should be treated in all patients, regardless of age. This decision, however, is both scientific and politic: the lower the criterion blood pressure, the greater the delivery system's need to absorb larger numbers of patients. Further complicating this decision is the finding that the elderly display the greatest variability in diastolic blood pressure, regardless of diagnostic and/or treatment status (14).

Added to the controversy surrounding compliance measurement is the fact that major inhibitors to compliant behavior remain. These can be summarized into: a) patient factors; b) prescribing habits of physicians; and c), provider/patient interaction.

Patient Factors

We are hampered by a lack of research specifically addressing compliance among aging patients. We do know that older persons are among the most health conscious and demonstrate disease preventive behaviors which are as adequate as in other age groups. These findings belie the generally perceived notion that the elderly are less reliable regarding disease preventive or health maintenance behavior. A self-fulfilling prophecy develops: since we expect less of this age group, we get less from them. The self-fulfilling prophecy can have unfortunate outcomes such as overly conservative treatment habits (24).

Sackett and Haynes (27) cite few patient-related demographic factors predictive of compliance. Of the 37 hypertension-related studies cited, 7 demonstrate compliance being positively associated with age while 30 demonstrate no association. While hypertension compliance research is not noted for its methodological rigor, it appears that being old is not a negative factor.

Potentially more predictive is research on patients' perceptions of medical situations. The best known of these is the Health Belief Model (3) which posits a series of interactive factors facilitating compliance. These include readiness to undertake compliant behaviors (e.g., general health motivations, willingness to accept medical direction, value of threat reduction, assessment of the probability that compliance will reduce threat) and a series of modifying (demographic, interactional, knowledge) and enabling factors.

While used frequently, the Health Belief Model is limited to disease avoidance and not compliance per se. Applications to chronic disease have met with limited success. Additionally, the model has an underlying clinical orientation: it accepts the physician's perspective that the patient will act in a highly rational manner. The Health Belief Model blames the patient for noncompliance. It contains predominantly patient characteristics; the physician is exonerated from blame.

A component of the Health Belief Model is the patient's level of knowledge about a medical condition since knowledge is a demonstrable prerequisite for compliance. Several studies have increased antihypertensive compliance through educational means (17,33). While the elderly see hypertension as more serious than do other age groups (22), only 32 percent of the population knew that hypertension was equivalent to high blood pressure. Worse yet, only 41 percent of the hypertensives knew that the two terms were equivalent. It is clear that education alone is inadequate to assure increased compliance. A more active approach is demanded.

The need for a more active patient role, the typically asymptomatic nature of hypertension, and the social location of older people suggest the use of blood pressure cuffs. If the patient is left alone to follow physician instructions, has minimal contact with and feedback from the provider, and has an asymptomatic condition, we are almost assuredly guaranteeing high failure rates. Most chronic diseases are "family affairs" or, at least, situations requiring interaction and role shifts among the patient and his/her significant others. In patients whose lifestyles are minimally affected by a condition such as hypertension, there is a need for the confluence of social support (30) and feedback on treatment progress. These principles were tested through the use of family- and self-monitored blood pressure cuffs and reported below.

The Prescribing Habits of Physicians

Avorn (1) asserts that medical schools have been "derelict" in providing geriatric pharmacologic information to their students, depending instead on pharmaceutical house "detail people." Avorn et al. (2) assert that clinicians' knowledge of several drugs is affected more by commercial messages than by scientific literature. Additionally, substantial evidence exists to indicate that clinicians dramatically overestimate the level of patient compliance (4,6,8) so that uncontrolled but treated hypertension results in increased dosage or prescription changes. A change has the potential for decreasing compliance in that the patient perceives the physician as groping for a solution to an asymptomatic problem. Changes in medication further exacerbate noncompliance by increasing the probability of side effects and self-medication errors and the monetary expense of staying well.

Physician/Patient Interaction

Documented as significantly causal of noncompliance is the nature of the relationship or interaction between patient and physician. Cassell (5) analyzes language used in clinical settings as influential in treatment outcome. The typically high emotional content of physician/patient interaction is not conducive to a relationship built on trust or to learning new behaviors. Both low and high anxiety situations are least productive of effective learning.

The "art" of medicine is, in part, the ability to establish an effective therapeutic relationship. Because communication is viewed as an "art," it is relegated to the genetic constitution of the clinician rather than seen as a learned behavior. Admission of noncompliance is viewed by patient and physician as patient failure and not within the clinician's medical domain. The dominant/submissive relationship assures that this behavior remains the patient's fault. It is necessary to recognize that the patient is responsible for his/her behavior. However, given the high rates of noncompliance reported in the literature, fault for noncompliance cannot rest wholly with the patient.

Factors in noncompliance do not seem to be related to drug side effects (9) even among the elderly (19). Instead, rank-ordered reasons given by patients for stopping medication are physicians telling them to stop, patients feeling that their blood pressure was normal, and feeling that they no longer needed treatment (13). Side effects and cost of treatment were far down the list. These reasons are related directly to the ability of the clinician to educate the patient about the nature of antihypertensive therapy. Whether or not the physician actually told the patients who stopped taking medication to do so is immaterial. Patients perceived this to be the case and the consequences of this perception are quite real.

Patients are more concerned with and, therefore, choose clinicians for interpersonal skills than for medical competence (7,25). Additionally, physicians misperceive by overestimating the extent to which patients desire involvement in their own therapy (32). Among the elderly, however, clinicians significantly <u>underestimated</u> their desire to participate, along with underestimating all patients' needs for information. Poor patient/physician communication with the elderly may result from factors such as: a) the older patient's inability to aggressively seek information; b) a higher level of health awareness and concern; and c) changing social roles. If we add to this the typically rushed nature of this interaction and inevitable personality and age differences, poor patient/physician communication seems almost inevitable.

While the cards seem stacked against this age group, dramatically positive changes have occurred. The next sections explore factors in compliance in older populations and new data related to motivating compliance through use of home blood pressure cuffs.

COMPLIANCE AMONG AGING PATIENTS

Attempts at other than pharmacologic reduction of blood pressure have been explored. However, it is difficult to maintain older patients on low salt and weight loss programs (11). While research on the relaxation response and biofeedback has been extensive, there is little evidence from controlled clinical trials to suggest either as a superior treatment modality (18). Furthermore, continuation of the relaxation response or biofeedback is also an adherence problem. Moser et al. (20) implore physicians to inform hypertensive patients that insurance companies assign equal actuarial survival probabilities to "controlled" hypertensives and normotensive insurees, and hence, equal insurance rates. This highly rational approach is, as seen earlier, a major difference between patient and physician.

We, therefore, must examine techniques for motivating compliance in older populations when standard, stepped, pharmacologic care is used. The HDFP investigations demonstrated that for persons 50 to 59 years of age, five-year death rates were 25.3 percent lower among those in stepped-care than those randomized into referred-care (31). For the population 60 to 69, five-year mortality was 16.4 percent lower in the stepped-care group. Thus, treatment convenience, the use of nonphysician personnel, and minimal side effects, (attributable to gradual medication increases), produced the greatest mortality reduction and, by implication, compliance.

Over time and without major motivational interventions, increasing numbers of older hypertensive patients bring their blood pressure under control. The 1973 and 1980 Minneapolis-St. Paul Community Surveys (10) demonstrate that among residents aged 55 to 59, the percentage of hypertensives under control increased dramatically. Furthermore, older individuals were less likely to be out of control than were younger persons. Similar results are found using self-report data: medication adherence is the same in young and old patients (23) while appointment keeping is better among older patients (19).

Since older patients do as well or better than younger patients in blood pressure reduction, can we determine a method which further enhances this capacity? Can we keep older patients in the system and thereby available for blood pressure reduction programs?

THE EXPERIMENTAL USE OF BLOOD PRESSURE CUFFS

Data were collected on 399 patients, aged 17 to 70, all with newly discovered hypertension (see Table 1). Patients were treated on identical stepped-care regimens at the Hypertension Specialty Clinic of the Indiana University School of Medicine by nurse practitioners under the supervision of physicians. The study's objective was to determine, in a controlled fashion, the best methodology for maintaining patients on antihypertensive therapy. Randomized groups using family-monitored blood pressure cuffs, self-monitored cuffs, and a control group on standard, stepped-care but no home cuff were compared for a period of up to six years. This study is published elsewhere (28). The use of either a self-monitored or family-monitored cuff is better than no cuff at maintaining patients on antihypertensive therapy for the first 18 months of treatment. The use of a family-monitored cuff produces substantial results in reducing drop-outs from the disease care delivery system for the first year of the study. No single methodology more effectively maintains patients at goal blood pressure or keeps them in the system over the long term. Since the use of cuffs better maintains patients in the system for about 18 months and since patients can't be treated unless they are in the system, we recommend the use of family-monitored or self-monitored cuffs where feasible.

The mean age in the study population is 47.4 years at entry and 29.8 percent are greater or equal to 55 years of age (N = 119); 61.7 percent (N = 246) are between 31 and 54. There is a statistically significant relationship (x^2 = 14.77;

df = 2; p < .001) between age and status in the system. At the conclusion of three years, 78.2 percent of those 55 and older remain in the system. The younger the patient, the more likely it is that he/she will drop out of the treatment. A drop-out refers to an individual not seen in the system for a period of one year and, therefore, includes those who have moved, died, or truly dropped out. Older patients are more motivated to maintain themselves in the system.

TABLE 1. Age and status in the system

Status	Age					
	16-30		31-54		55 and older	
	N	%	N	%	N	%
Active	16	47.1	153	62.2	93	78.2
Drop-out	18	52.9	93	37.8	26	21.8
Total	34	100.0	246	100.0	119	100.0

Remaining active in the system may be attributable to the influence of a family member. There is an inverse linear relationship between age and the patient's ability, upon inquiry, to identify a "significant other" available to take the patient's blood pressure. Despite this relationship, no statistically significant differences, regarding continuing in the system, exist between the patients with and those without a family member. The presence of a family member for motivating patient continuity is less important than the patient's age. The older the patient, the more likely it is that he/she will remain in the disease care delivery system (Table 2).

Since age and system continuity are related, is it possible to further enhance this relationship with the methods tested here? For those using family-monitored cuffs, 95.8 percent of the older patients stayed in treatment (compared with 68.1 percent of those aged 31-54 and 50 percent of the patients less than 31; $x^2 = 9.47$; df = 2; p < .01). For the self-monitored group, 79.5 percent of those 55 or older stayed in treatment, compared to 64.2 and 38.5 percent of the middle-aged and young, respectively ($x^2 = 7.79$; df = 2; p < .05). There was no relationship between age and system continuity for the control group. Older patients are better able to maintain themselves in the system with the added feedback from a blood pressure cuff, either family-monitored or self-monitored.

The key question is whether the elderly achieve better blood pressure control than do younger patients. To answer this question, goal diastolic blood pressure is used. For persons aged 30 or less, the mean diastolic blood pressure for all clinic visits in a 6-month period had to be less than or equal to 90 mm Hg to be at goal. Persons aged 31 and over are considered at goal if their mean diastolic blood pressure for a 6-month period is less than or equal to 95 mm Hg. While this

TABLE 2. Motivational intervention by age and status in the system

	Age					
	16-30		31-54		55 and older	
Status	N	%	N	%	N	%
Family-read Cuff						
Active	4	50.0	32	68.1	23	95.8
Drop-out	4	50.0	15	31.9	1	4.2
Total	8	100.0	47	100.0	24	100.0
Self-read Cuff						
Active	5	38.5	61	64.2	31	79.5
Drop-out	8	61.5	34	35.8	8	20.5
Total	13	100.0	95	100.0	39	100.0
Control						
Active	7	53.8	60	57.7	39	69.6
Drop-out	6	46.2	44	42.3	17	30.4
Total	13	100.0	104	100.0	56	100.0

criterion denies the importance of systolic hypertension, it does provide a rough, age-graded measure of blood pressure control. The most dramatic differences are between the youngest patients and both of the other age groups, early in the course of the study (Table 3). During the first 12 months of treatment, significantly fewer young patients are at goal blood pressure than in the other 2 groups. In the first 6 months of treatment, 37.5 percent of the youngest group were at goal while 58.3 and 56.6 percent of the middle and oldest groups, respectively, were at goal.

In all but the first six-month period, the oldest group had the greatest proportion at goal blood pressure while the youngest group had the smallest proportion. Even using the more liberal goal criterion of the two older groups for the youngest group did not change the results of this analysis. Several conclusions are suggested. First, it takes the older patients somewhat longer to achieve a clinically desired goal

TABLE 3. Percent of patients at goal blood pressure by age and duration in study

	Age					
Duration in	16-30		31-54		55 and older	
Study (months)	N	%	N	%	N	%
0 - 6	12	37.5	137	58.3[a]	64	56.6[a]
7 - 12	13	46.4	130	65.3[a]	72	71.3[a]
13 - 18	12	57.1	121	67.6[a]	76	79.2[a]
19 - 24	10	58.8[b]	110	67.5[b]	66	74.2[b]

[a] $p < .05$ as compared to 16-34 age group.
[b] $p < .03$ as compared to 55 and older age group.

blood pressure. Second, once achieved, and despite the typically more complex medical regimens for older people, they perform no worse than the middle-aged population (aged 31-54) and clearly far better than the youngest group. And finally, the youngest group not only drops out of the system more readily, but for those remaining in the system, poorer compliance is obtained. Data beyond the two years presented show no differences.

Which intervention is most effective for the various age groups? For patients using family-monitored blood pressure cuffs, a greater percentage of the oldest patients were at goal than for the other two age groups (see Table 4). However, none of the differences in the percentages at goal by age group for any time period were statistically significant. Using self-monitored blood pressure cuffs produced the most consistently beneficial results for the oldest age group.

TABLE 4. Percent at goal and difference tests by intervention and time period, for patients 55 and older

Time Period (months)	Blood pressure group	N	Percent at Goal
0 - 6	Family-monitored	23	82.6
	Self-monitored	35	68.6[a]
	Control	55	38.2[b]
7 - 12	Family-monitored	23	60.9[c]
	Self-monitored	32	90.6
	Control	46	63.0[d]

[a] $p < .0003$ as compared to family-monitored
[b] $p < .003$ as compared to self-monitored
[c] $p < .005$ as compared to self-monitored
[d] $p < .004$ as compared to self-monitored

Although only a few of the comparisons were statistically significant, the oldest age group using the self-monitored blood pressure cuff consistently had more of its patients at goal than either of the other age groups. These results ranged from a low of 68.6 percent at goal during the first 6 months to a high of 90.6 percent at goal for the 7-12 month period. The control group demonstrated mixed results. Those over 55 were less consistently at goal than the other age groups. However, with time, they tended to catch up in the percent at goal blood pressure. Using a self-monitored, and to a lesser degree, family-monitored cuff has the beneficial effect of most quickly bringing the newly diagnosed hypertensive under control. Not only are the elderly more likely to stay in the delivery system, but they seem to respond the best to the various motivational interventions used here.

Finally, it is important to know which, if any, of the motivational interventions is most effective for the oldest cohort at specific time periods. This knowledge is needed for getting the elderly under control as quickly as possible, and for keeping them in the system and under control for as long as possible. Tests for the differences of proportions at goal are used at each time period. For the critical first six months, either motivational intervention is superior to standard treatment of newly discovered hypertension. Therefore, for older patients able to read a mercury monometer and hear the first and fifth Korotkoff sounds, or with an available significant other, the loan or purchase of a blood pressure cuff will facilitate achieving goal blood pressure.

Curiously, and contrary to theoretical expectations, during the next six-month period, patients with self-monitoring cuffs are more likely to be at goal than either the control group or those with a family-monitored cuff. Following the first full year of treatment, there are no statistically significant differences between either of the interventions or the control group in keeping persons age 55 and over at goal blood pressure. Those in the control group appear to catch up. The use of the blood pressure cuffs, either family-monitored or self-monitored, are beneficial in keeping older patients in the system and in bringing newly discovered hypertension quickly under control. Long-term benefit derived from the cuffs is not indicated by these data.

CONCLUSIONS AND IMPLICATIONS

Older patients are more likely to be compliant with antihypertensive regimens than are younger patients. They are concerned about their health and threats to their longevity. Additionally, Medicare enhances the likelihood of seeking medical care. Therefore, hypertension has a high probability of being detected, treated, and controlled in this age group. Of particular concern when treating hypertension is keeping the patient in the disease care delivery system. Patients using publicly funded clinics, with their potential for episodic care, are most likely to drop out of treatment. Therefore, a major objective for physicians treating hypertension must be maintaining the individual in the delivery setting. The research reported here demonstrates that older, newly discovered hypertensive patients using self-monitored or family-monitored blood pressure cuffs can be kept in the system for up to 18 months. This is a critical time as it is the first step in assuring long-term control. Patients with family-monitored blood pressure cuffs are most likely to remain in treatment. Having family members involved in the patient's blood pressure assessment is a motivational reminder for medication taking. Self-monitored cuffs are almost as effective at system continuity as family-monitored cuffs while both are better than standard clinic treatment.

While it took longer for older patients to reach goal blood pressure, once achieved, maintenance at goal was better than in other age groups. Again, the use of either type of cuff more effectively facilitated maintenance at goal than no cuff. Therefore, the use of cuffs should be based on the availability of a significant other and the patient's visual and auditory acuity.

Once a patient commits to controlling his/her hypertension by returning for regular check-ups, approximately 75 percent of all patients stay at goal, with or without the use of a blood pressure cuff. While there is a slight edge in control to family-monitored cuffs, it appears that over time, patients who remain in the system will have their blood pressure brought under control. Unfortunately, we do not know if patients lost to followup dropped out because their blood pressure was not controlled quickly.

Remaining in the system seems to be the most critical variable. Blood pressure cuffs have their greatest impact, not in the long run, but in providing the patient with information that motivates return early in treatment. Therefore, aggressive medical treatment, coupled with a blood pressure cuff used by the patient in his/her home, is likely to result in significant success in blood pressure reduction for this age group. Older patients are more compliant; inability to control their hypertension is more likely to be a therapeutic than a compliance problem. Despite warnings of impaired eyesight and hearing and problems associated with the complexity of taking multiple tablets at variable intervals, achievement of blood pressure control in older, inner-city residents is quite possible.

If we are correct in asserting that the physician/patient encounter is anxiety-provoking, making learning difficult--and instruction on medication compliance is learning--then we must look for additional learning sites. The pharmacy profession has begun recently to assert its central role in patient education. Unfortunately, patients perceive that the majority of treatment information comes from physicians with only a minor amount from pharmacists (13). Not only must pharmacists educate patients more aggressively about medication, they must be able to educate patients about the pharmacist's role as educators. This profession has yet to convince the public of its role in patient education. Given their vast and detailed knowledge, this gap represents an unfortunate information loss in the system for the patient.

Hypertension, unlike a cerebrovascular accident, is a condition of insufficient drama for the mobilization of social support systems facilitative of compliance. The blood pressure cuff provides some of that awareness, especially when family members are involved. The more "public" the statement of a behavioral intention, and the use of a cuff is just that, the greater the probability of a correspondence between intention and behavior.

REFERENCES

1. Avorn, J. (1983): Health Affairs, 2:23-32.
2. Avorn, J., Chen, M., and Hartley, R. (1982): Am. J. Med., 73:4-8.
3. Becker, M.H. (1976): In: Compliance with Therapeutic Regimens, edited by D.L. Sackett and R.B. Haynes, pp. 40-50. Johns Hopkins University Press, Baltimore.
4. Caron, H.S., and Roth. H.P. (1968): JAMA, 203:120-124.
5. Cassell, E.J. (1985): Talking with Patients. The Theory of Doctor-Patient Communication, Vol. 1. MIT Press, Cambridge, Massachusetts.
6. Chobanian, A.V. (1980): In: Patient Compliance to Prescribed Antihypertensive Medication Regimens: A Report of the National Heart, Lung, and Blood Institute, NIH Pub. No. 81-2101, edited by R.B. Haynes, M.E. Mattson, and T.O. Engebretson, Jr., pp. xi-xii. Bethesda, Maryland.
7. Congalton, A.A. (1969): Med. J. Aust., 24:1165.
8. DiMatteo, M.R., and DiNicola, D.D. (1982): Achieving Patient Compliance. The Psychology of the Medical Practitioner's Role. Pergamon Press, New York.
9. Fitzgerald, J.D. (1976): In: Compliance with Therapeutic Regimens, edited by D.L. Sackett and R.B. Haynes, pp. 119-128. Johns Hopkins University Press, Baltimore.
10. Folsom, A.R., Loepker, R.V., Gillum, R.F., Jacobs, D.R., Prineas, R.J., Taylor, H.L., and Blackburn, H. (1983): JAMA, 250:916-921.
11. Franklin, S.S. (1983): Med. Clin. North Am., 67:395-417.
12. Fries, J.F. (1980): N. Engl. J. Med., 303:130-135.
13. Haines, C.M., and Ward, G.W. (1981): Public Health Rep., 96:514-522.
14. Hypertension Detection and Follow-up Program Cooperative Group (1979): JAMA, 242:2562-2571.
15. Kasl, S.V. (1984): Am. Heart J., 108:660-669.
16. Koch, H. (1983): National Center for Health Statistics Advance Data, 89:1-11.
17. Levine, D.M., Green, L.W., Deeds, S.G., Chwalow, J., Russell, R.P., and Finlay, J. (1979): JAMA, 241:1700-1703.
18. McCann, B.S. (1986): In: Progress in Behavioral Modification, edited by M. Hersen, R.M. Eisler, and P.M. Miller, in press. Academic Press, New York.
19. Morisky, D.E., Levine, D.M., Green, L.W., and Smith, C.R. (1982): Arch. Intern. Med., 142:1835-1838.
20. Moser, M., Rafter, J., and Gajewski, J. (1984): JAMA, 251:756-757.

21. National Heart, Lung, and Blood Institute (1973): The Public and High Blood Pressure. D.H.E.W. Pub. No. (NIH) 77-356. Washington, D.C.
22. National Heart, Lung, and Blood Institute (1981): The Public and High Blood Pressure. Six Year Follow-up Survey of Public Knowledge and Reported Behavior. NIH Pub. No. 81-2118. Bethesda, Maryland.
23. Nelson, E.C., Stason, W.B., Neutra, R.R., and Solomon, H.S. (1980): Prev. Med., 9:504-517.
24. O'Malley, K., and O'Brien, E. (1980): N. Engl. J. Med., 302:1397-1401.
25. Poole, A.D., and Sanson-Fisher, R.W. (1979): Soc. Sci. Med., 13A:37-43.
26. Rowland, M., and Roberts, J. (1982): National Center for Health Statistics Advance Data, 84:1-10.
27. Sackett, D.L., and Haynes, R.B., editors (1976): Compliance with Therapeutic Regimens. Johns Hopkins University Press, Baltimore, Maryland.
28. Stahl, S.M., Kelley, C.R., Neill, P.J., Grim, C.E., and Mamlin, J. (1984): Am. J. Public Health, 74:704-709.
29. Stahl, S.M., Lawrie, T., Neill, P., and Kelley, C. (1977): Am. J. Public Health, 67:345-352.
30. Stahl, S.M., and Potts, M.K. (1985): In: Social Bonds in Later Life. Aging and Interdependence, edited by W.A. Peterson and J. Quadagno, pp. 305-323. Sage Publications, Beverly Hills, California.
31. Stamler, R. (1983): Prev. Med., 12:155-162.
32. Strull, W.M., Lo, B., and Charles, G. (1984): JAMA, 252:2990-2994.
33. Swain, M.A., and Steckel, S.B. (1981): Res. Nurs. Health, 4:213-222.
34. Veterans Administration Cooperative Study Group on Antihypertensive Agents (1967): JAMA, 202:1028-1034.
35. Veterans Administration Cooperative Study Group on Antihypertensive Agents (1970): JAMA, 213:1143-1152.

ALCOHOL CONSUMPTION, BLOOD PRESSURE, AND AGING:
RESULTS FROM THE NORMATIVE AGING STUDY

Robert J. Glynn, Glen R. Bouchard, and John A. Hermos*

Normative Aging Study, Veterans Administration
Outpatient Clinic, and Boston University
School of Public Health, Boston, Massachusetts 02108;
*Department of Medicine and Surgery,
Veterans Administration Medical Center, and
Department of Medicine, Boston University School of Medicine,
Boston, Massachusetts 02130

Several epidemiologic studies have found a relationship between heavier alcohol consumption and elevated blood pressure (3,11,12,14,20,26-28,34). This relationship exists in diverse adult populations and remains strong when such potentially confounding variables as sex, body mass, and cigarette smoking are considered. Conclusions drawn by these studies include that alcohol may be the most prevalent cause of reversible hypertension (25). Specifically, if the relationship between alcohol consumption and blood pressure is causal, then about one third of the cases of hypertension among individuals drinking three or more drinks per day would be due to alcohol consumption (15). Estimates from an Australian study (28) are that 11 percent of hypertension in men and 1 percent in women are attributable to drinking, assuming the relationship is causal.

There are several reasons why the effects of alcohol consumption on blood pressure may differ or be particularly important in the elderly. Systolic blood pressure levels in developed countries tend to increase with age so that even if the effect of heavier drinking were uniform across age, elderly heavier drinkers would be at greater risk of the adverse effects of high blood pressure. Older individuals have proportionally less lean tissue and alcohol is not fat soluble so that equal quantities of alcohol may affect an older person more than a younger one. Vogel-Sprott and Barrett (36) found the amount of impairment in task performance induced by administration of a fixed dose of alcohol to increase greatly with age. The elderly are more likely to be taking medications and are, thus, more prone to drug-alcohol interactions.

Drinking behaviors developed over a lifetime may also be more difficult to moderate in newly diagnosed elderly hypertensives. This chapter discusses the epidemiologic evidence for the relationship between drinking and blood pressure and the way this relationship may change with age. Results from previous studies are compared with drinking and blood pressure data from the Normative Aging Study, a longitudinal study of human aging. The possibility that the relationship is causal and due to a pressor or withdrawal effect of alcohol consumption on blood pressure is contrasted to the possibility that the relationship is artifactual and due to the personality or physiology of individuals choosing to be heavier drinkers. Finally, we discuss the possibility of altering drinking behaviors in the elderly and whether alcohol-related hypertension is reversible.

NORMATIVE AGING STUDY

The Normative Aging Study is a longitudinal study of aging initiated in 1963 and located at the Veterans Administration Outpatient Clinic in Boston (5). Participants were recruited through radio and newspaper advertisements and by appeals to companies whose employees were likely to remain in the Boston area (e.g., insurance companies and local police and fire departments). Volunteers were screened at entry according to health criteria in order to provide a population initially free of known chronic medical conditions. In particular, volunteers were excluded from participation if they had a history or a finding upon examination of such conditions as hypertension, heart disease, diabetes, cancer, cirrhosis, pancreatitis, peptic ulcer, gout, or recurrent asthma, bronchitis, or sinusitis. Alcohol consumption and alcohol-related problems were not among the screening criteria, but several of the disqualifying conditions mentioned above are related to heavy alcohol use. Many alcoholics have no medical complications and, thus, would not have been excluded.

With these criteria, the study enrolled 2,280 community-dwelling men born between 1884 and 1945. Fourteen percent of these men had less than a high school education, 25 percent were high school graduates, 35 percent went beyond high school, and 26 percent were college graduates. The study protocol calls for these participants to report for physical examinations every five years if they are less than 52 years old; after their 52nd birthday, they report every three years. At each examination, blood pressure is measured by an examining physician using a standard mercury sphygmomanometer with a 14 cm cuff. With the subject seated, systolic blood pressure and fifth-phase diastolic blood pressure are measured once in each arm to the nearest 2 mm Hg. The palpatory method is used to check auscultatory systolic readings. Blood pressure has been assessed by this same methodology since the inception of the study. Further details about the Normative Aging Study population and the study protocol are available elsewhere (6). The population for the present report is the 1,955 male participants in the Normative Aging Study who were born after 1891 and were still participating in the study in September 1982. At that time, the Normative Aging Study mailed a 15-page drinking questionnaire to these men. Completed questionnaires were returned by 1,713 men. This instrument was a revised version of a drinking questionnaire mailed to this population in 1973 (18). For each of 16 distinct alcoholic beverages, respondents were asked to record the average number of drinks of each they were currently consuming per day, per week, per month or per year. Average alcohol consumption, measured in drinks per year, was estimated for each respondent to be the total number of drinks of all types. All beverages were considered together because, according to the U.S. Department of Agriculture (1), 12 ounces of beer, 5 ounces of table wine, and 1.5 ounces of distilled spirits all contain approximately 0.60 ounces of absolute alcohol. Respondents were asked to give the number of days in a typical month on which they consumed seven or more drinks. This gives some measure of periodic or regular heavier drinking. The questionnaire contained 13 items asking about current effects of drinking. We classified respondents as drinkers with problems if they reported that alcohol was regularly affecting their physical health or psychosocial functioning. Specifically, respondents were identified as drinkers with problems if they reported any of the following effects of drinking during the past year: a) once or more a month--"I got drunk too often, I felt sick upon awakening, I had memory lapses or blackouts, I had the shakes, I became hostile, it made me more depressed, I hurt myself physically when drunk, it affected my health, it affected my family relationships"; or b) once or more a week--"I had difficulty sleeping, I was skipping meals." In addition, respondents were classified as drinkers with problems if they had been arrested for drunken driving, or for drunkenness and disturbing the peace at least once during the preceding year. The questionnaire also asked respondents to report the frequency and dosage of all prescription and over-the-counter medications they had taken for more than a month during the past year. Medications were coded according to the American Hospital Formulary Service (30). Men were classified as taking antihypertensive medications if they were taking diuretics (code 40:28), hypotensive agents (code 24:08), or certain cardiac drugs (code 24:04) with hypotensive properties (beta blockers or calcium channel blockers).

Of the 1,955 men in the population for the current report, 1,681 had at least one regularly scheduled Normative Aging Study physical examination between January 1978 and March 1985. Of the 274 unexamined men, 144 were participating in the study only by answering mailed questionnaires, in many cases because they had moved away from the Boston area; the remaining 130 unexamined men did not report for scheduled physical examinations. One thousand, five hundred and fifty men both completed the 1982 drinking questionnaire and had a physical examination since 1978. Comparing participation rates across three 18-year birth cohorts (born 1892-1909, born 1910-1927, and born 1928-1945) men in the middle cohort were about twice as likely as men in the oldest and youngest cohort to both report for a physical examination and respond to the drinking questionnaire. Men who reported for a physical examination since 1978, but did not respond to the 1982 drinking questionnaire, had systolic and diastolic blood pressure levels similar to those of questionnaire respondents. Men who responded to the drinking questionnaire, but have not reported for a physical examination since 1978, had slightly but not significantly lower average alcohol consumption levels compared to men who reported for a physical examination between January 1978 and March 1985. Results reported in this paper are based on the 1,550 men who both answered the 1982 drinking questionnaire and had a physical examination between January 1978 and March 1985.

Analyses, in this chapter, relate blood pressure measurements from a participant's most recent physical since 1978 to measures of drinking and usage of antihypertensive medications assessed in the 1982 questionnaire. Body weight and current cigarette consumption levels, considered to be potential confounders, were assessed at the physical examinations. There is some misclassification bias due to the differences in timing between the sets of measures. Fifty-nine percent of the blood pressure assessments occurred in 1981, 1982, or 1983 and so were only one year removed from the administration of the drinking questionnaire; 89 percent of blood pressure assessments occurred during the years 1980-1984. There is some evidence that drinking behaviors in older men are fairly stable over time (17) and this limits the misclassification bias.

To assess possible age differences in the relation between alcohol consumption behaviors and blood pressure, we partitioned the population into three 18-year birth cohorts: men born 1892-1909, born 1910-1927, and born 1928-1945. The effects of aging on systolic and diastolic blood pressure within each birth cohort were assessed using analysis of covariance (33,35) to adjust for blood pressure levels at entry into the Normative Aging Study. Analysis of covariance was also used to assess the cohort-specific relationship of drinking behaviors with systolic and diastolic blood pressure, controlling for body mass index, smoking, and age. Data from men taking blood pressure lowering medications and men not taking such medications were analyzed separately.

Aging and Blood Pressure

Systolic blood pressure levels are known to rise with age in developed countries. Diastolic pressure levels rise until about age 56, then decline thereafter (24). These relationships may differ in non-Western societies (29). Table 1 shows the percentage of men within three birth cohorts in the Normative Aging Study who reported on their 1982 drinking questionnaires that they were taking blood pressure lowering medications. Since the protocol of the Normative Aging Study required these men to be normotensive upon entry into the study (between 1963 and 1970), this table gives a measure of the age-specific cumulative incidence of hypertension from entry into the study until September 1982. There were no significant differences among cohorts in mean followup time. Rates of medication usage were similar in the two oldest cohorts but much lower in the youngest cohort. Part of the difference between cohorts in medication rates could be due to a hesitancy to introduce lifelong drug therapy in the youngest cohort. The lack of differences between the two oldest cohorts may be the result of uncertainty about the benefits of drug therapy in the elderly hypertensive (2).

TABLE 1. Reported usage of blood pressure altering medications in 1982 within three birth cohorts

Birth year	Medications			
	no	%	yes	%
1892-1909	59	79	16	21
1910-1927	727	77	214	23
1928-1945	467	87	67	13
Total	1253	81	297	19

Chi-square = 23.1, degrees of freedom = 2, $p < 0.001$.

Adjusted mean changes in blood pressure levels within birth cohorts from entry into the Normative Aging Study until the participant's most recent examination between January 1978 and March 1985 are shown in Tables 2 and 3. Means are adjusted for initial levels because blood pressure readings show a marked tendency for regression to the mean (19). Table 2 presents mean changes for men not reporting usage of blood pressure lowering medications on their 1982 drinking questionnaire. Over an interval averaging 16.5 years, men in the two oldest cohorts had much greater rises in systolic blood pressure than men in the youngest cohort. Systolic blood pressure levels actually declined longitudinally on average among men in the youngest cohort not taking hypotensive drugs. Rate of change in systolic blood pressure over time was clearly not uniform across age groups--a finding similar to that of Rabkin et al. (32). Diastolic blood pressure levels had the opposite trend

TABLE 2. Change of blood pressure levels[a]

Birth year	N	Examination 1963-1970	1978-1985
1892-1909	59	8.78 ± 1.81[b]	-3.35 ± 1.04
1910-1927	727	5.48 ± 0.51	-0.56 ± 0.30
1928-1945	467	-1.21 ± 0.64	0.40 ± 0.37
		F = 38.6, p < 0.001	F = 6.47, p = 0.002

[a]From entry examination (1963-1970) to most recent Normative Aging Study examination (1978-1985); men not taking blood pressure, medications at followup.
[b]Mean ± S.E.M. systolic blood pressure.

over time in this group. Men in the oldest cohort had a decline over time of 3.4 mm Hg in adjusted diastolic levels, whereas mean changes in diastolic level among men in the other two cohorts were less than 1 mm Hg.

Data in Table 3 are from men reporting usage of hypotensive medications on their 1982 drinking questionnaire. Trends for substantial increases in systolic blood pressure levels and for declines in diastolic levels among older men are similar to those in Table 2. These differences among treated men are difficult to interpret because selection for treatment and the aggressiveness of blood pressure therapy may differ across age groups (2).

TABLE 3. Change in blood pressure levels[a]

Birth year	N	Examination 1963-1970	1978-1985
1892-1909	16	5.58 ± 3.71[b]	-6.21 ± 2.24
1910-1927	214	4.95 ± 1.02	-1.08 ± 0.61
1928-1945	67	1.18 ± 1.84	2.86 ± 1.11
		F = 1.68, p = 0.19	F = 8.34, p < 0.001

[a]From entry examination (1963-1970) to most recent Normative Aging Study examination (1978-1985); men taking blood pressure, medications at followup.
[b]Mean ± S.E.M. systolic blood pressure.

Alcohol Consumption Behaviors and Blood Pressure

The relationship of the current average annual alcohol consumption, in September 1982, with blood pressure in each of the three cohorts was first examined using three categorical measures of elevated blood pressure. Based on chi-square tests (Tables 4-6), there were no significant differences in any of the cohorts between alcohol consumption in the percentages of men with systolic blood pressure of 140 mm Hg or greater, diastolic blood pressure of 90 mm Hg or greater, or the percentage of men taking hypotensive medications. Although roughly descriptive of group differences, these chi-square tests are insensitive to trends in rates with heavier beverage consumption. In the two younger cohorts, which include a substantial number of men (Tables 5 and 6), the percentages of men with elevated systolic blood pressure were highest among men drinking 1-3 drinks per day and men drinking 3 or more drinks per day. In these two youngest cohorts, nondrinkers had the lowest percentage of men taking hypotensive medications. The percentage of men in the youngest cohort drinking at least three drinks per day, who had elevated systolic blood pressures, was more than twice the percentage among men in this cohort drinking less than one drink per day.

TABLE 4. Percent of men born 1892-1909 with elevated blood pressure within five alcohol consumption groups

Drinks/year	N	% Systolic bp $\geq$ 140	% Diastolic bp $\geq$ 90	% Taking bp medications
none	17	18	0	18
1-29	8	50	13	0
30-364	28	39	11	21
365-1094	19	26	0	37
$\geq$ 1095	3	67	0	0
		Chi-square = 5.3 $p = 0.26$	Chi-square = 4.6 $p = 0.33$	Chi-square = 5.8 $p = 0.21$

Comparing Tables 4-6, there were substantial differences across cohorts in alcohol consumption levels. In the oldest cohort (Table 4), 3 of the 75 men (4 percent) drank 3 or more drinks per day, whereas 25 men (33 percent) drank less than 30 drinks per year. In the cohort born 1910-1927, 13 percent drank 3 or more drinks per day, 21 percent drank less than 30 drinks per year; and in the cohort born 1928-1945, 17 percent drank at least 3 drinks per day, 13 percent drank less than 30 drinks per year.

TABLE 5. Percent of men born 1910-1927 with elevated blood pressure within five alcohol consumption groups

Drinks/year	N	% Systolic bp $\geq$ 140	% Diastolic bp $\geq$ 90	% Taking bp medications
none	129	22	7	18
1-29	66	23	8	24
30-364	414	22	8	24
365-1094	210	29	9	24
$\geq$ 1095	122	28	4	21
		Chi-square = 4.2 $p = 0.38$	Chi-square = 2.5 $p = 0.65$	Chi-square = 2.5 $p = 0.65$

TABLE 6. Percent of men born 1928-1945 with elevated blood pressure within five alcohol consumption groups

Drinks/year	N	% Systolic bp ≥ 140	% Diastolic bp ≥ 90	% Taking bp medications
None	53	8	6	8
1-29	16	6	19	13
30-364	248	9	8	15
365-1094	125	11	10	10
≥ 1095	92	18	10	13
		Chi-square = 7.5 p = 0.11	Chi-square = 3.3 p = 0.51	Chi-square = 3.5 p = 0.48

Tables 7-9 present cohort-specific adjusted mean levels of systolic blood pressure within medication groups and alcohol consumption groups. These means were adjusted for body mass index, birth year, and cigarette smoking status, which are known factors to be related to blood pressure (26), and may differ across alcohol consumption groups. Similar adjusted means for diastolic levels were estimated. The differences between alcohol consumption groups in mean diastolic levels were insubstantial and results are not presented.

TABLE 7. Adjusted mean levels of systolic blood pressure within alcohol consumption groups for men born 1892-1909

Drinks/year	N	No medication	N	Medication
None	14	127.0 ± 5.0[a]	3	141.1 ± 12.2
1-29	8	134.6 ± 6.4	0	
30-364	22	139.3 ± 3.9	6	143.1 ± 8.4
365-1094	12	132.3 ± 5.4	7	124.3 ± 8.1
≥ 1095	3	151.6 ± 11.5	0	
		F = 1.54, p = 0.20 Trend chi-square = 2.5 p = 0.12		F = 1.31, p = 0.31 Trend chi-square = 1.07 p = 0.32

[a]Mean ± S.E.M. systolic blood pressure.

Among men in the oldest cohort, who were not taking hypotensive medications (Table 7), there was some tendency for regular alcohol users to have higher systolic blood pressures; but the small number of men in this cohort, drinking three or more drinks per day, precluded a reliable estimation of group-specific means. There were also too few men in this cohort taking medications lowering their blood pressure to be able to estimate the effects of alcohol consumption in the medicated group.

The cohort of men, born 1910-1927, is of ample size to reasonably estimate the effects of alcohol consumption in both the medicated and nonmedicated groups (Table 8). Among men in this cohort not taking hypotensive medications, the adjusted mean systolic blood pressure level in the men drinking three or more drinks per day was slightly higher (from 1.6 to 3.2 mm Hg) than mean levels in other alcohol consumption groups. Differences among the adjusted means in the alcohol consumption groups were not significant nor was there convincing evidence for an increasing trend in systolic levels across heavier consumption groups. Among men in this cohort taking hypotensive medications, the adjusted mean systolic levels were substantially higher in the two highest alcohol consumption groups. Men in these two groups had adjusted mean systolic levels between 8.1 and 10.8 mm Hg higher than the adjusted means of the men in the two groups drinking less than 30 drinks per year. Evidence for a linear trend of increasing systolic levels across heavier alcohol consumption groups was strong.

TABLE 8. Adjusted mean levels of systolic blood pressure within alcohol consumption groups for men born 1910-1927

Drinks/year	N	No medication	N	Medication
None	106	128.7 ± 1.5[a]	23	127.9 ± 3.0
1-29	50	127.1 ± 2.1	16	128.5 ± 3.6
30-364	316	127.5 ± 0.8	98	133.2 ± 1.5
365-1094	159	127.5 ± 1.2	51	138.7 ± 2.0
≥ 1095	96	130.3 ± 1.5	26	136.6 ± 2.9
		$F = 0.78, p = 0.54$		$F = 3.15, p = 0.02$
		trend chi-square = 0.3		trend chi-square = 10.1
		$p = 0.61$		$p = 0.002$

[a]Mean $\pm$ S.E.M. systolic blood pressure.

Among men in the cohort born 1928-1945, who were not taking hypotensive medications, the pattern of adjusted mean systolic levels was similar but slightly more pronounced than that among men in the adjacent cohort (Table 9). Men drinking three or more drinks per day had adjusted mean systolic levels between 2.9 and 5.5 mm Hg higher than the means of men in other alcohol consumption groups. Although differences in adjusted mean systolic levels were small among men in the four groups drinking less than three drinks per day, the test for linear trend was significant. Among men in the youngest cohort taking hypotensive medications, there were too few men drinking less than 30 drinks per year to allow for meaningful estimation of adjusted group means.

TABLE 9. Adjusted mean levels of systolic blood pressure within alcohol consumption groups for men born 1928-1945

Drinks/year	N	No Medication	N	Medication
None	49	120.0 + 1.9[a]	4	120.8 + 8.4
1-29	15	119.0 + 3.5	1	134.3 + 11.9
30-364	226	120.0 + 0.9	22	126.3 + 2.7
365-1094	111	121.6 + 1.2	14	133.4 + 4.8
≥ 1095	75	124.5 ± 1.5	17	132.8 ± 4.8
		$F = 1.9$, $p = 0.11$		$F = 0.9$, $p = 0.47$
		Trend chi-square = 5.3		Trend chi-square = 2.4
		$p = 0.02$		$p = 0.13$

[a]Mean ± S.E.M. systolic blood pressure.

Because small numbers in some cells precluded reliable estimation of some group means, and because there were no clear differences across cohorts in the relationship of drinking and systolic blood pressure, another regression model was used to estimate group differences in all cohorts combined. Results for men not taking hypotensive medications are shown in Table 10 which also includes estimates of the effects of birth year, body mass index, and cigarette smoking. Adjusted mean systolic levels in each of these four groups were estimated to be between 3.1 and 3.8 mm Hg lower than the level of men drinking three or more drinks per day. T-tests for the significance of

TABLE 10. Regression of systolic blood pressure on alcohol consumption groups, birth year, body mass index, and cigarette smoking status for men not taking blood pressure medications

Variable	Regression coefficient	Standard error	p-value
Nondrinker vs ≥ 3 drinks/day	-3.4	1.6	0.03
0-29 drinks/year vs ≥ 3 drinks/day	-3.8	2.0	0.06
30-364 drinks/year vs ≥ 3 drinks/day	-3.4	1.3	0.01
1-3 drinks/day vs ≥ 3 drinks/day	-3.1	1.4	0.03
Birth year (minus 1900)	-0.49	0.049	0.01
Body mass index (kg/m^2)	0.83	0.13	0.01
Current cigarette smoker (1 = yes, 0 = no)	-1.9	1.1	0.06
Intercept	119.1		

R-square = 0.108
F test for drinking groups = 2.1, $p = 0.08$
Chi-square for trend with drinking groups = 4.0, $p = 0.05$

these differences have p-values between 0.01 and 0.06. Although the test for linear trend was significant, differences between adjusted mean systolic levels among men in the first four drinking groups were no more than 0.7 mm Hg. There was virtually no effect of consuming up to three drinks per day on systolic blood pressure levels of men not taking hypotensive medications.

For men taking hypotensive medications, estimated mean systolic blood pressure differences, between light and nondrinkers and men drinking three or more drinks per day, were much larger than among untreated men (Table 11). Standard errors of estimated effects in this table were much larger than in Table 10, mostly because of the smaller number of treated men. In this group, the mean systolic level for men drinking between one and three drinks per day was very similar to the mean among men drinking three or more drinks per day. Nondrinkers had adjusted mean systolic levels 8.8 mm Hg lower, and men drinking between one and three drinks per day had adjusted mean systolic levels only 0.2 mm Hg lower, compared to men drinking three or more drinks per day. Evidence for a linear association of alcohol consumption with systolic blood pressure was much stronger in men taking hypotensive medications.

TABLE 11. Regression of systolic blood pressure on alcohol consumption, birth year, body mass index, and cigarette smoking status for men taking blood pressure medications

Variable	Regression coefficient	Standard error	p-value
Nondrinker vs ≥ 3 drinks/day	-8.8	3.8	0.02
0-29 drinks/year vs ≥ 3 drinks/day	-6.8	4.5	0.13
30-364 drinks/year vs ≥ 3 drinks/day	-4.3	2.8	0.14
1-3 drinks/day vs ≥ 3 drinks/day	-0.2	3.1	0.95
Birth year (minus 1900)	-0.48	0.13	0.01
Body mass index (kg/m^2)	0.67	0.25	0.01
Current cigarette smoker (1 = yes, 0 = no)	-1.7	2.6	0.50
Intercept	128.7		

R-square = 0.090
F test for drinking groups = 2.4, p = 0.05
Chi-square for trend with drinking groups = 9.1, p = 0.003

Mean daily consumption is only one measure of alcohol consumption and certain problematic drinking behaviors can be masked unless variability of consumption and the effects of drinking are considered. Table 12 shows the adjusted mean systolic blood pressure levels within groups defined by the number of days in a typical month on which seven or more drinks were consumed. Among men not taking hypotensive medications, the adjusted mean systolic level was markedly higher among men consuming seven or more drinks a day, about twice a week or more often. There was no substantial difference in adjusted mean systolic levels among the three groups of men not drinking seven or more drinks in a day at least eight times per month.

TABLE 12. Adjusted mean levels of systolic blood pressure within groups defined by the number of days in a month drinking seven or more drinks

Frequency	N	No medication	N	Medication
Nondrinkers	169	125.2 ± 1.1[a]	30	127.3 ± 2.8
Drink, but not 7 drinks in a day	787	125.2 ± 0.5	200	133.0 ± 1.1
1-7 days/month	193	126.4 ± 1.1	42	131.9 ± 2.4
≥8 days/month	87	130.1 ± 1.6	20	139.0 ± 3.5
		$F = 2.9, p = 0.03$		$F = 2.4, p = 0.07$
		trend chi-square = 5.9		trend chi-square = 4.2
		$p = 0.02$		$p = 0.04$

[a]Mean $\pm$ S.E.M. for systolic blood pressure.

Among men taking blood pressure lowering medications, the effect of drinking seven or more drinks in a day, about twice a week or more often, was more pronounced. These men had adjusted mean systolic levels 11.7 mm Hg more than nondrinkers and 6.0 mm Hg more than drinkers who did not drink seven or more drinks in a day. Notable here is the far lower adjusted mean systolic level among nondrinkers compared to all drinkers.

Table 13 presents adjusted mean systolic levels for men who reported that alcohol was currently adversely affecting their physical, psychological, or social functioning, compared to men with no such problems. Self-reported drinking problems made little difference in the adjusted mean systolic levels of men not taking hypotensive medications. Among men taking hypotensive medications, those reporting problems with drinking had adjusted mean systolic levels 6.0 mm Hg higher than the adjusted mean level of men not reporting problems. As with average daily consumption and periodic heavy drinking days, problems with drinking had the strongest association with the systolic blood pressure levels of men taking hypotensive medications.

TABLE 13. Adjusted mean levels of systolic blood pressure for men reporting problems with drinking and men reporting no problems

Reported problems with drinking	N	No medication	N	Medication
no	1111	125.6 + 0.4[a]	257	132.9 + 1.0
yes	142	127.1 ± 1.2	40	138.9 ± 2.5
		F = 1.3, p = 0.25		F = 6.7, p = 0.01

[a]Mean ± S.E.M. for systolic blood pressure.

CONCLUSIONS

Results from the Normative Aging Study are in conformity with results from several other populations in finding higher mean systolic blood pressure levels among men drinking three or more drinks per day (3,11,12,14,20,26-28,34). Most of these studies found men drinking less than three drinks per day to have slightly higher mean systolic levels, compared to nondrinkers, but these differences were quite small. Participants in the Normative Aging Study, drinking less than three drinks per day and not taking hypotensive medications, had mean systolic blood pressure levels almost identical to nondrinkers. Criqui et al. (12) found that treated hypertensives tended to be heavier drinkers than both untreated hypertensives and normotensives. A new finding in the present data is that the influence of drinking on systolic blood pressure levels may be much greater among men taking hypotensive medications, and that among these men, even one or two drinks per day may have a substantial impact. Periodic heavy drinking and problems with drinking also had a much stronger effect on treated men. It is unclear whether this is due to enhanced responsivity to alcohol among hypertensives, to a drug-alcohol interaction, or to lower compliance with drug regimens among heavier drinkers.

In the Normative Aging Study data, there was no evidence for a different association of drinking with systolic blood pressure levels among different birth cohorts. In the two cohorts with substantial numbers of men, associations were similar for both treated and untreated men. Fortmann et al. (14) found a stronger association between drinking and systolic blood pressure among men aged 50-74 than among men aged 20-49. By contrast, Criqui et al. (12) found no association between drinking and blood pressure among men over age 50 drinking less than 30 ml per day of alcohol (about two drinks).

It is possible that the elderly are somewhat protected from the adverse effects of heavier drinking because they tend to drink less than younger people. Compared to the younger, the elderly have a higher percentage of nondrinkers and fewer heavy and problem drinkers (10). Longitudinal drinking data from the

Normative Aging Study suggest that cross-sectional age differences in drinking behaviors may be more attributable to cohort differences or period effects than to true aging effects (17). Over a nine year period from 1973 to 1982, there were no substantial declines in cohort-specific mean alcohol consumption levels or in rates of drinking problems. If future generations of the elderly drink more, then higher rates of alcohol-induced illnesses can be expected among that age group.

The association of alcohol consumption with blood pressure, observed in a cross-sectional study, is difficult to interpret because elevated blood pressure may affect drinking behaviors. There have been only a few longitudinal studies of drinking and the development of hypertension. Dyer et al. (13) reported that problem drinkers, from the Chicago Peoples Gas Company, compared to nonproblem drinkers, and men from the Chicago Western Electric Company, drinking more than six drinks per day compared to men drinking less, had markedly higher incidences of hypertension over four years and a much greater increase in both systolic and diastolic blood pressures. The Framingham Study (20) reported that participants who increased their drinking had slight increases in both systolic and diastolic blood pressure; those who decreased their drinking had slight decreases in both systolic and diastolic blood pressure. In the Normative Aging Study, men drinking three or more drinks per day had incidence rates of hypertension about 1.6 times more than those of nondrinkers (7).

In nonalcoholics, evidence on the acute effects of alcohol on blood pressure is conflicting (31,37). Potter and Beevers (31) did find evidence for a pressor effect of alcohol on blood pressure among hypertensives. They followed 16 hypertensive men who regularly drank up to 80 g of alcohol daily. In a controlled hospital environment, they found that when these men abstained from alcohol, their blood pressures declined and remained lower; when drinking resumed, blood pressure levels rose markedly and remained high. This provides further reason to suspect that alcohol may have a greater effect on hypertensive men. In addition to a direct pressor effect, a withdrawal effect of alcohol on blood pressure has been described. Alcoholics undergoing detoxification, experience blood pressure rises as they go through withdrawal (9,34). It has been proposed that the elevated systolic blood pressure levels observed in population studies may be partly attributable to subclinical manifestations of alcohol withdrawal because participants have typically reported after an overnight fast (37). It is also possible that the association of higher blood pressure with heavier alcohol consumption is partly due to a "selection effect" because men prone to higher blood pressures are more likely to choose to drink more heavily. Multivariate analyses, controlling for potential confounding variables, attempt to adjust for this possibility, but some variables, such as underlying personality traits, cannot be adequately controlled.

The clinical significance of alcohol-induced hypertension is unclear. There is a substantial amount of evidence that moderate alcohol consumption may protect against coronary heart disease (22). Friedman et al. (16) followed two matched groups of 850 hypertensive patients each for 12 years; one group reported drinking at least three alcoholic drinks per day per person, and the other group reported drinking fewer than three drinks per day. The two groups had similar frequencies of cardiovascular complications leading to hospitalization or death, except for coronary disease for which alcohol may be protective. Two recent studies indicate that not all hypertension is equally malignant (4,8). Hypertensive men with low body mass indices had higher mortality rates than hypertensive men with high body mass indices. Whether alcohol-induced hypertension carries the same risk for mortality as hypertension among light and nondrinking individuals, is not known.

Moderation of heavier drinking is recommended for newly diagnosed hypertensives. At least for some individuals, the onset of disease leads to spontaneous changes in drinking behaviors (23). However, the modification of drinking behaviors is no simple task. Kaplan (25) described the poor long-term success rate of weight reduction programs for hypertensives. Drinking behaviors, like eating behaviors, are very complex (18) and may be equally difficult to modify. Alcoholics are known to have low long-term success rates in abstaining from drinking or reducing to moderate drinking (21). Long-term success rates for drinking reduction in nonalcoholic populations have not been studied.

In summary, aging in Western societies is associated with rises in blood pressure for many individuals. Heavier drinking (three or more drinks per day) has been found in several studies to be correlated with elevated systolic blood pressure levels. This relationship persists, even in controlling for known confounding variables such as body mass, age and smoking. Among men in the Normative Aging Study, similar effects of drinking on systolic blood pressure were found in men of different ages. In men not taking hypotensive medications, those drinking three or more drinks per day had mean systolic blood pressure levels (adjusted for age, body mass index, and cigarette smoking) 3.4 mm Hg higher than nondrinkers (95 percent confidence interval: 0.3-6.5 mm Hg). In men taking hypotensive medications, those drinking three or more drinks per day had adjusted mean systolic blood pressure levels 8.8 mm Hg higher than nondrinkers (95 percent confidence interval: 1.4-16.2 mm Hg). Reported problems with drinking and periodic heavier drinking (drinking seven or more drinks on some days in a typical month) were also related to elevated systolic levels. Therefore, the greater effect of heavier drinking on hypertensive men has three interpretations: 1) there may be a group of men whose blood pressures are very reactive to heavier drinking; 2) alcohol may affect the action of antihypertensive medications; and 3) heavier drinkers may be less compliant with taking medications.

ACKNOWLEDGMENTS

Supported by the Medical Research Service of the Veterans Administration and by Grant No. AA06739 from the National Institute on Alcohol Abuse and Alcoholism.

REFERENCES

1. Adams, C.F. (1975): Nutritive Values of American Foods in Common Units. Agriculture Research Service Agricultural Handbook No. 456. US Govt. Printing Office, Washington, DC.
2. Amery, A., Birkenhager, W., Brixko, P., Bulpitt, C., Clement, D., Deruyterre, M., De Schaepdryver, A., Dollery, C., Fagard, R., Forette, F., Forte, J., Hamdy, R., Henry, J.F., Joossens, J.V., Leonetti, G., Lund-Johassen, P., O'Mally, K., Petrie, J., Strasser, T., and Tuomilehto, J. (1985): Lancet i:1349-1354.
3. Arkwright, P.D., Belin, L.J., Rouse, I., Armstrong, B.K., and Vandongen, R. (1982): Circulation, 66:60-66.
4. Barrett-Connor, E., and Khaw, K.-T. (1985): Circulation, 72:53-60.
5. Bell, B., Rose, C.L., and Damon, A. (1972): Aging Human Dev., 3:5-17.
6. Bosse', R., Ekerdt, D.J., and Silbert, J.E. (1984): In: Handbook of Longitudinal Research: Teenage and Adult Cohorts, Vol. 2, edited by S.A. Mednick, M. Harway, and K.M. Finello, pp. 273-289. Praeger Scientific, New York.
7. Bouchard, G., Conway, C., Hermos, J., and Glynn, R. (1984): Gerontologist, 24(Suppl.):259 (Abstract).
8. Cambien, F., Chretien, J.M., Ducimetiere, P., Guize, L., and Richard, J.L. (1985): Am. J. Epidemiol., 122:434-442.
9. Clark, L.T., and Friedman, H.S. (1985): Alcoholism: Clin. Exp. Res., 9:125-130.
10. Clark, W.B., and Midanik, L. (1982): In: Alcohol Consumption and Related Problems. Alcohol and Health Monograph No. 1, pp. 3-52, National Institute on Alcohol Abuse and Alcoholism, Rockville, Maryland.
11. Cooke, K.M., Frost, G.W., and Stokes, G.S. (1983): Clin. Exper. Pharmacol. Physiol., 10:229-233.
12. Criqui, M.H., Wallace, R.B. Mishkel, M., Barrett-Connor, E., Heiss, G. (1981): Hypertension, 3:557-565.

13. Dyer, A.R., Stamler, J., Paul, O., Berkson, D., Shekelle, R., Lepper, M.H., McKean, H., Lindberg, H.A., Garside, D., and Tokich, T. (1981): Circulation, 64(Suppl. III): 20-27.
14. Fortmann, S.P., Haskell, W.L., Vranizan, K., Brown, B.W., and Farquhar, J.W. (1983): Am. J. Epidemiol., 118:497-507.
15. Friedman, G.D., Klatsky, A.L., and Siegelaub, A.B. (1982): Hypertension, 4:143-150.
16. Friedman, G.D., Klatsky, A.L., and Siegelaub, A.B. (1983): Ann. Intern. Med., 98:846-849.
17. Glynn, R.J., Bouchard, G.R., LoCastro, J.S., and Laird, N.M. (1985): Am. J. Public Health, (in press).
18. Glynn, R.J., LoCastro, J.S., Hermos, J.A., and Bosse, R. (1983): J. Stud. Alcohol, 44:1011-1025.
19. Glynn, R.J., Rosner, B., and Silbert, J.E. (1982): Circulation, 66:724-731.
20. Gordon, T., and Kannel, W.B. (1983): Arch. Intern. Med., 143:1366-1374.
21. Helzer, J.E., Robins, L.N., Taylor, J.R., Carey, K., Miller, R.H., Combs-Orme, T., and Farmer, A. (1985): N. Engl. J. Med., 312:1678-1682.
22. Hennekens, C.H. (1983): In: Prevention of Coronary Heart Disease, edited by N.M. Kaplan, and J. Stamler, pp. 130-138. W.B. Saunders, Philadelphia, Pennsylvania.
23. Hermos, J.A., LoCastro, J.S., Bouchard, G.R., and Glynn, R.J. (1984): In: Nature and Extent of Alcohol Problems Among the Elderly, edited by G. Maddox, L.N. Robins, and N. Rosenberg, pp. 117-132. National Institute on Alcohol Abuse and Alcoholism, Rockville, Maryland.
24. Kannel, W.B., and Gordon, T. (1978): Bull. N.Y. Acad. Med., 54:573-591.
25. Kaplan, N.M. (1985): Ann. Intern. Med., 102:359-373.
26. Klatsky, A.L., Friedman, G.D., Siegelaub, A.B., and Gerard, M.J. (1977): N. Engl. J. Med., 296:1194-1198.
27. Kozarevic, D., Racic, Z., Gordon, T., Kaelber, C.T., McGee, D., and Zukel, W.J. (1982): Am. J. Epidemiol., 116:287-301.
28. MacMahon, S.W., Blacket, R.B., MacDonald, G.J., and Hall, W. (1984): Hypertension, 2:85-91.
29. Maddocks, I. (1961): Lancet ii:396-399.
30. McEvoy, G.K., editor (1983): American Hospital Formulary Service. American Society of Hospital Pharmacists, Bethesda, Maryland.
31. Potter, J.F., and Beevers, D.G. (1984): Lancet i:119-122.
32. Rabkin, S.W., Mathewson, F.A.L., and Tate, R. (1979): Am. J. Epidemiol., 109:650-662.
33. SAS Institute, Inc. (1982): SAS User's Guide: Statistics. SAS Institute, Cary, North Carolina.
34. Saunders, J.B., Beevers, D.G., and Paton, A. (1981): Lancet ii:653-656.

35. Seber, G.A.F. (1977): Linear Regression Analysis. John Wiley, New York.
36. Vogel-Sprott, M., and Barrett, P. (1984): J. Stud. Alcohol, 45:517-521.
37. Wallace, R.B., Lynch, C.F., Pomerhn, P.R., Criqui, M.H., and Heiss, G. (1981): Circulation, 64(Suppl. III):41-47.

PHENYLETHANOLAMINE N-METHYLTRANSFERASE IN NORMAL AND ALZHEIMER'S DISEASE BRAINS

William J. Burke,*[†] Hyung D. Chung,*[†] Randy Strong,*[†] Gary L. Marshall,* J. Wendell Davis,[†] and Tong H. Joh**

*Veterans Administration Medical Center and [†]St. Louis University School of Medicine, St. Louis, Missouri 63125; and **Cornell University Medical College, New York, New York 10021

Using a recently developed specific and highly sensitive assay for phenylethanolamine N-methyltransferase (PNMT), the marker for the neurotransmitter, epinephrine, we have found evidence for this transmitter in human cortex. In addition, we have found a significant decrease in the activity of the epinephrine-forming enzyme in the locus coeruleus and cortical areas of an Alzheimer's disease brain. Immunocytochemical staining of locus coeruleus and rostral ventral lateral medulla (C-1) and rostral dorsal medial medulla (C-2) regions for PNMT, using PNMT antibodies and the peroxidase-antiperoxidase technique, revealed a decrease in PNMT positive axonal projections to the locus coeruleus in the Alzheimer's disease brain. The number of neurons in the locus coeruleus were also decreased in the Alzheimer's disease brain. However, PNMT positive neuronal cell bodies in C-1 and C-2 regions were not significantly decreased in the Alzheimer compared to the control. Atrophy was, however, noted in some C-1 and C-2 neurons from the Alzheimer's disease case. These results suggest that changes in PNMT in C-1 and C-2 axonal projections to locus coeruleus and cortical neurons were retrograde, secondary to loss of postsynaptic locus coeruleus and cortical neurons and were not due to primary loss of PNMT neurons in C-1 and C-2 regions. The results indicate that the epinephrine neuronal system may be affected in Alzheimer's disease and suggest that retrograde transsynaptic atrophy may play an important role in loss of neuronal function in Alzheimer's disease. The significance of these findings to future therapeutic strategies is discussed.

METHODS FOR LOCALIZING BRAIN PNMT

PNMT Assay

PNMT is the terminal enzyme in the catecholamine biosynthetic pathway, where it catalyzes the transfer of a methyl group from S-adenosyl-L-methionine (SAM) to norepinephrine to form epinephrine. Bulbring (10) first demonstrated the methylation of norepinephrine to epinephrine in the adrenal gland where PNMT is present in high concentration (11,12). Axelrod (5) purified the enzyme from adrenal gland and developed a widely used [^{3}H]SAM-based assay for adrenal PNMT. Knowledge of the importance of PNMT in various tissues has grown with development of more sensitive assays.

The original assays did not have sufficient sensitivity to locate PNMT in the brain and investigators thought that it was found only in the adrenal gland. Saaverda's modification (58) increased the sensitivity of the assay by 50-fold and by using this, PNMT could be found in the brain. Other brain PNMT assays were developed using high pressure liquid chromatography with electrochemical detection (hplc-ec) to separate and quantitate epinephrine formed by the enzyme (8,63). These assays were reported to have a sensitivity of 0.3 to 0.5 picomoles. Specificity of the assay was improved by using the natural substrate, norepinephrine, rather than phenylethanolamine and measuring epinephrine as the product of the reaction. Both radiochemical and hplc-ec methods demonstrated PNMT in the locus coeruleus and other brainstem nuclei as well as hypothalamus, basal ganglia, and spinal cord of the human central nervous system (35,37,47,63). However, even the most sensitive of these methods (35,47) did not detect PNMT in specific regions of human cerebral cortex. We have recently developed a highly sensitive and specific radiochemical PNMT assay (13) which uses norepinephrine and [^{14}C]SAM as substrates and measures the natural product, epinephrine. Nonspecific methyltransferases (57) do not interfere with this assay which has a sensitivity of 0.03 picomoles. In addition, use of dialysis instead of dilution to remove enzyme inhibitors allows reduction of the homogenizing volume by one fifth that previously used, giving the assay an overall sensitivity 50 times that of previous assays. The increased sensitivity of this assay allows measurement of PNMT in specific regions of human cerebral cortex (Table 1) not previously shown to contain the enzyme (35,47).

Immunocytochemical Localization of PNMT

Besides the [^{3}H]SAM-based enzyme assays, immunohistochemical methods have been used to localize the PNMT neuronal system in the central nervous system (4,29-31,55). These methods have used specific antibodies to PNMT protein and anti-immunoglobulin antibodies conjugated with peroxidase to stain specifically PNMT-containing neurons and axon terminals (4,30,55,62). In rats, immunohistochemical techniques have been used to localize one group of PNMT neurons in the C-1 region, and a second smaller group in the C-2 region (29,31). The axon terminals of these PNMT neurons project onto norepinephrine neurons in the locus coeruleus, and onto other neurons in brainstem nuclei, the hypothalamus, and spinal cord (4,29-31,55).

TABLE 1. PNMT activity in various regions of human brain[a]

Brain region	PNMT activity (pmole/hr/gl)
Frontal (middle frontal gyrus)	31.8 + 5.17
Amygdala	58.1 ∓ 0.66
Hippocampus	32.5 ∓ 0.61
Parietal (angular gyrus)	35.5 ∓ 1.73
Occipital (area 18)	28.7 ∓ 1.48
Cerebellum (posterior inferior)	30.3 ∓ 1.29
Cerebellum (anterior superior)	33.9 ∓ 0.92
Choroid plexus	5.7 ± 0.19

[a]PNMT activity was measured in dialyzed supernatant from autopsy brain (control case #5) in regions where it had not been previously detected in man. A PNMT assay previously described was used to measure enzyme activity (see text). Each mean (+ SE) is derived from two replicate assays.

The capacity of antisera from one species to cross-react with the same enzyme from other species has allowed localization of other catecholamine-forming enzymes (e.g., tyrosine hydroxylase) in a variety of species including man. For this, antiserum to the enzymes from bovine adrenal (32) or human pheochromocytoma tissue has been used (49,50). This capacity of antisera to enzyme from one species to cross-react with the enzyme from other species has been attributed to the highly conserved structure of the enzyme molecule between species (32). Although several studies have used immunocytochemical techniques to localize tyrosine hydroxylase, the initial enzyme in catecholamine biosynthesis in human brain (32,52), there has been no previous immunocytochemical localization of PNMT in human brain.

PNMT IN NORMAL HUMAN BRAIN

Kopp et al. (35) reported human brain PNMT activity in C-1 and C-2 neurons as well as in their axonal projection areas: the locus coeruleus, periaqueductal grey, hypothalamus, and basal ganglia. However, neither Kopp et al. (35) nor Nagatsu et al. (47) found significant PNMT in the cerebral or cerebellar cortex, hippocampus, or amygdala. On the other hand, Mefford et al. (45) noted the presence of small amounts of epinephrine, the product of PNMT, in the human cortex, hippocampus, and amygdala. Using our recently developed assay (13), we have shown the presence of PNMT in frontal, parietal, occipital, and cerebellar areas of the human cortex as well as in the hippocampus, amygdala, and choroid plexus (Table 1). The PNMT activity in these areas was from 2 percent to 20 percent of that found in the locus coeruleus. The results indicate a wider distribution and suggest greater functional importance for PNMT than was previously known. The fact that PNMT is found in areas of the brain where its product, epinephrine, is present indicates that PNMT is a marker for this neurotransmitter. Inasmuch as it is the final enzyme in the catecholamine biosynthetic pathway, PNMT is a specific marker for epinephrine neurons and axon terminals.

We have used immunocytochemical staining (4,55,62) with antibody to bovine PNMT (32) to localize this enzyme in the human brain. The specificity of this method is demonstrated by the fact that locus coeruleus neurons, which are known to contain both tyrosine hydroxylase and dopamine beta-hydroxylase, enzymes with homology to PNMT, do not stain immunocytochemically using PNMT antibody (Fig. 1). PNMT positive neurons are seen in the C-1 (Fig. 2), as well as C-2 (our unpublished observation) regions of human brain. PNMT stained axonal projections are seen adjacent to both locus coeruleus neurons as well as blood vessels (Fig. 1). The data in Table 1 also note PNMT activity associated with brain blood vessels of the choroid plexus. Potential epinephrine receptors of the beta adrenergic type were found in the locus coeruleus, Table 2 (14,18). The fact that the 41 percent decrease in beta receptors was less than expected compared to the 89.5 percent decrease in the number of neurons in the Alzheimer's disease

TABLE 2. Beta receptors, PNMT activity, and neuronal density in locus coeruleus from a control and an Alzheimer patient[a]

Group	Beta receptors (fmole/mg protein)	PNMT activity (pmole/hr/g)	LC neuron density (neurons/field)
Control	40.9 + 1.72	376 + 15	95 + 2.12
Alzheimer	24.3 ∓ 1.16[b]	97 ∓ 0.16[b]	10 ∓ 1.5[b]

[a]Beta receptors, PNMT, and number of neurons were measured in the locus coeruleus from control #5 and Alzheimer's disease #2. Receptors and PNMT were measured according to previously described methods (see text). Locus coeruleus neurons were counted in three comparable haematoxylineosin stained sections in areas of maximum cell density. Each mean ($\pm$ SE) is derived from three replicate assays.
[b]$p < 0.005$ compared to control.

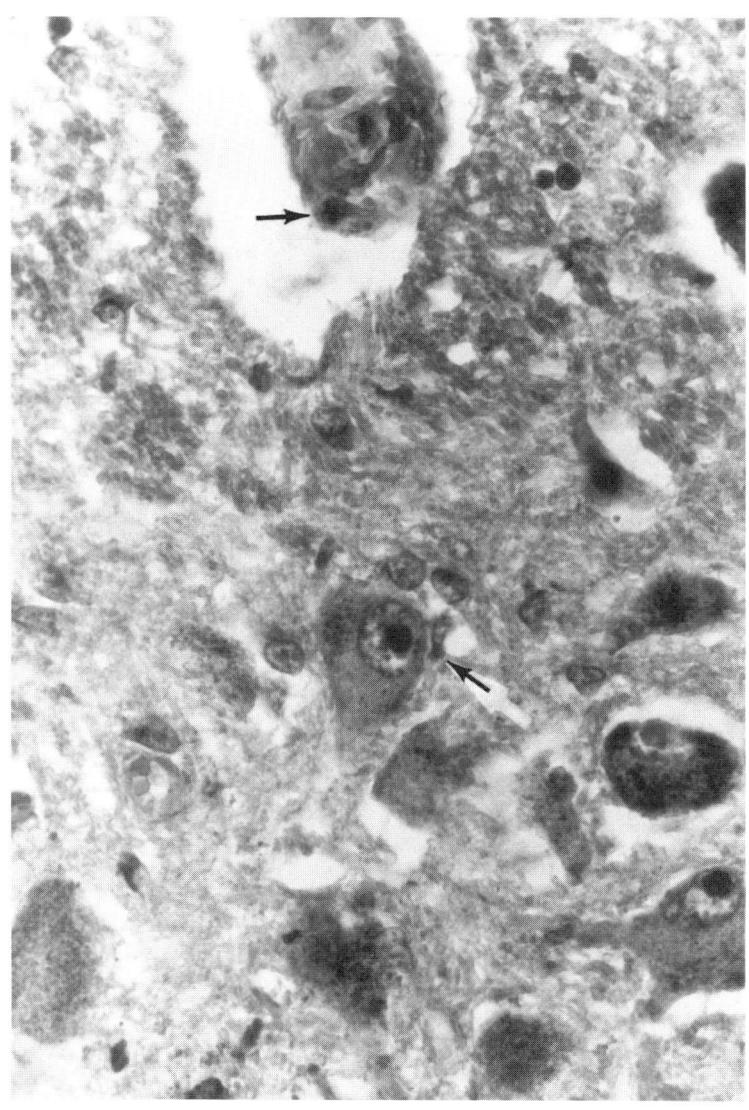

FIG. 1(A). Locus coeruleus neurons and blood vessels with adjacent PNMT positive axons from control case #6 (A) and Alzheimer case #2 (B and C). Comparable sections through the locus coeruleus from a control and an Alzheimer patient were stained immunohistochemically with PNMT antibody (see text). Arrows indicate PNMT positive axons. Magnification 125x.

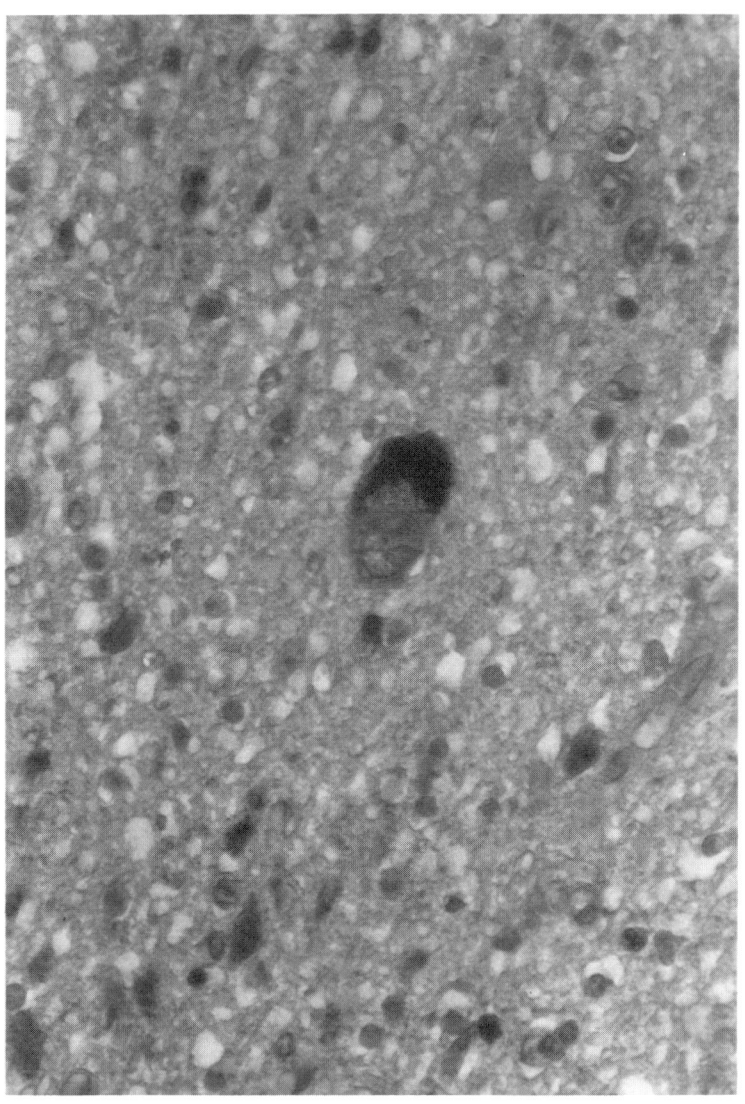

FIG. 1(B). See Fig. 1(A) legend.

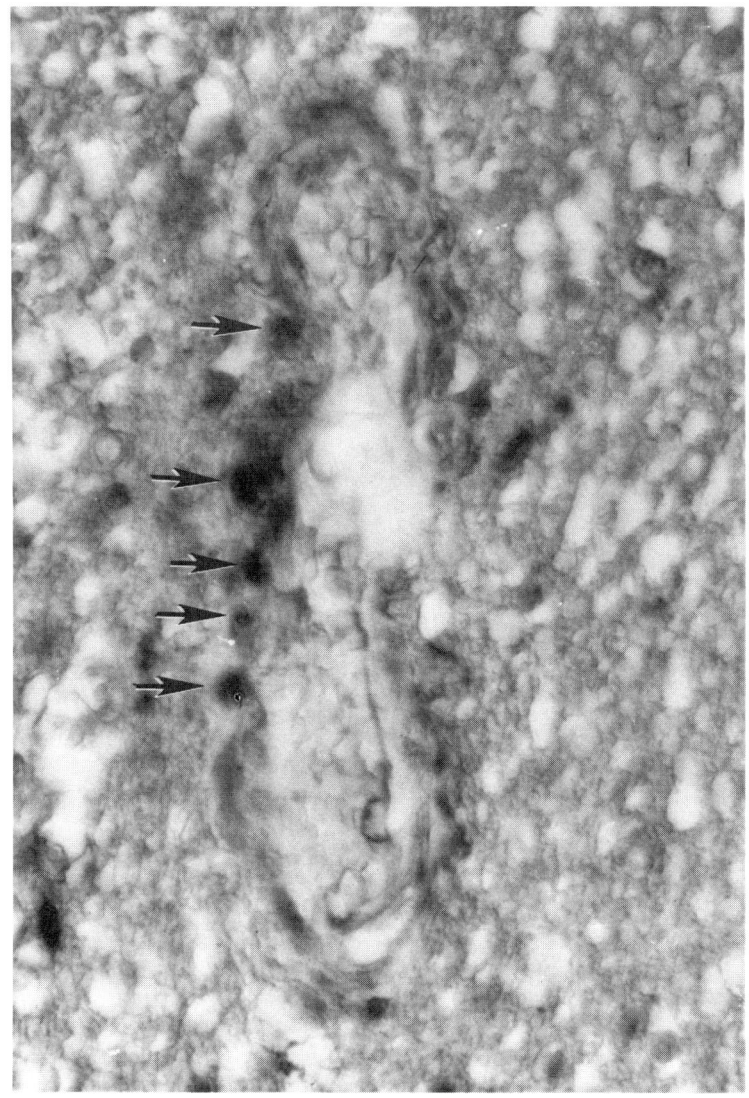

FIG. 1(C). See Fig. 1(A) legend.

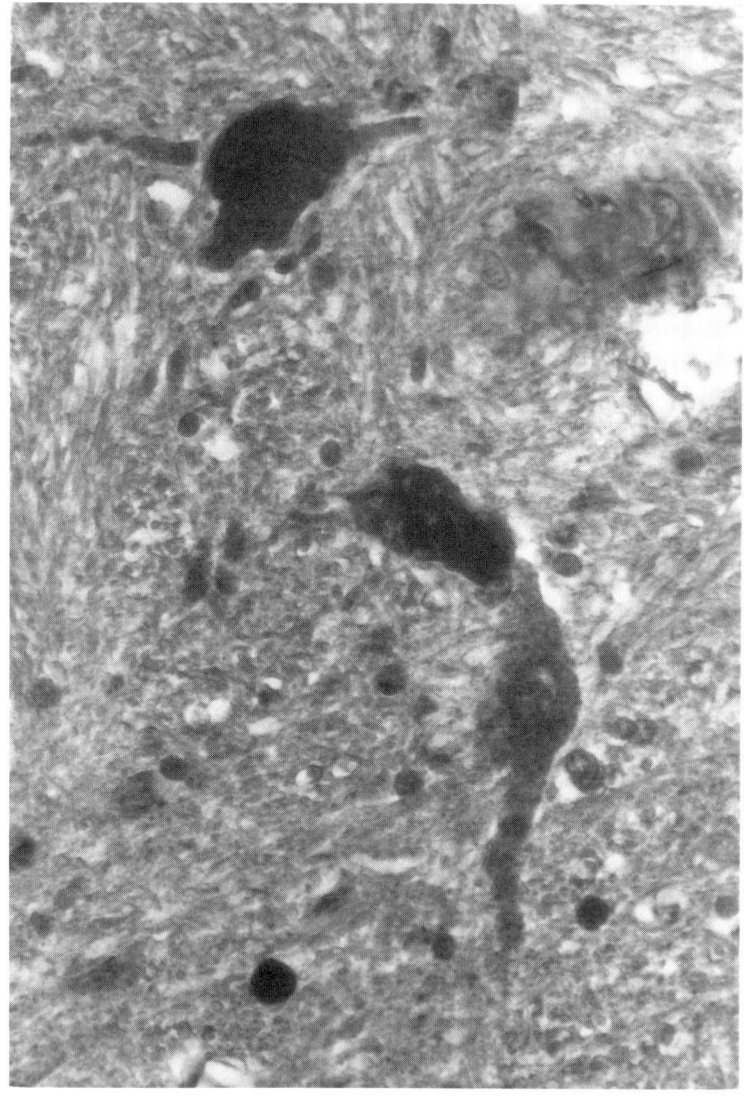

FIG. 2(A). C-1 neurons from control case #6 (A) and Alzheimer case #2 (B). Comparable sections through the C-1 region from a control and an Alzheimer patient were stained immunohistochemically with PNMT antibody (see text). Arrows indicate atrophic neurons. Magnification 125x.

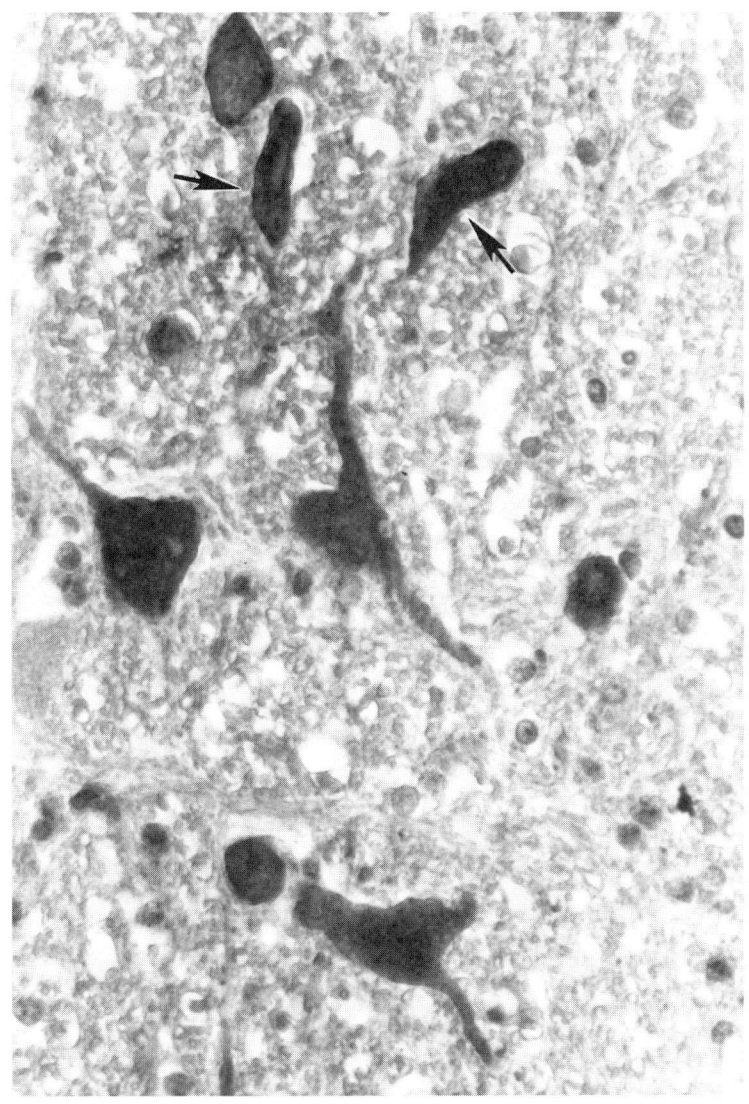

FIG. 2(B). See Fig. 2(A) legend.

case suggests that there was either a compensatory increase in beta receptors in Alzheimer's disease or that some of the receptors may be associated with blood vessels. These results are in accord with the possibility that epinephrine neurons in the C-1 and C-2 regions may influence locus coeruleus neurons, directly and indirectly, through alterations in the microvascular circulation of this region.

PNMT IN ALZHEIMER'S DISEASE

Although there has been an isolated report of PNMT activity in the brains of sufferers of Alzheimer's disease (63), no thorough study has been done. We have examined PNMT in detail in several areas of the brain from control and Alzheimer patients. The diagnosis of Alzheimer's disease in all cases was based on the clinical history as well as pathological findings of neurofibrillary tangles and senile plaques (Fig. 3) (16,24). The data of Table 3 and 4 show a diminution of 84 percent in PNMT activity in the locus coeruleus and from 65 percent to 76 percent in cortical areas from Alzheimer's disease brains compared to controls (Tables 3 and 4).

To determine whether differences in PNMT activities could be due to loss of enzyme, secondary to pre- or postmortem factors, (3,9,42,43,44), a number of control cases were examined. Table 5 lists some premortem factors which were considered. The clinical diagnoses in the Alzheimer cases were similar to those found in control cases, with the exception of Alzheimer's disease and its manifestations. Although control case #6 had a clinical diagnosis of dementia, the subject's mental status seemed to fluctuate with his overall medical condition and no pathology was found in the brain at autopsy. The age of controls ranged from 40 to 79 years which encompassed the ages of the Alzheimer cases. Control #1 had significant hypoxia (PO_2 < 40 mm Hg) unresponsive to treatment for three days prior to death. Normal PNMT levels in the brain of this subject indicate that prolonged hypoxia is not a factor in reducing PNMT levels. Medications used in the Alzheimer group, including a beta blocker and a cardiac glycoside, were also used by various members in the control group. A cholinergic agonist in one Alzheimer's disease patient was used topically in doses which would not be expected to affect brain function. Dexamethasone, a drug known to affect PNMT levels (11,12), was used in control #4; however, it had no effect on the locus coeruleus PNMT. The length of coma experienced prior to death ranged from 0.5 hours to 4 days. Since control #6 had the longest period of coma and the lowest locus coeruleus PNMT among the controls, coma duration may affect PNMT. The considerably shorter periods of coma in the Alzheimer cases compared to this control indicate the lower PNMT in an Alzheimer subject was not, per se, the result of coma.

TABLE 3. PNMT activity in locus coeruleus of control and Alzheimer patients[a]

Group	Age (years)	Cause of death	Death--refrig. (minutes)	Death--autopsy (hour)	Autopsy--assay (days)	PNMT activity
Control 1	68	Pneumonia	60	22.6	2	297 ± 2.2
Control 2	63	Cardiac arrest	220	20	47	306 ± 9.5
Control 3	40	Pneumonia	57	21.6	29	275 ± 4.1
Control 4	58	Cardiac arrest	120	14	8	313 ± 10.8
Control 5	69	Cardiac arrest	45	13.2	13	376 ± 15
Control 6	79	Cardiac arrest	180	17.5	137	193 ± 3.3
Alzheimer 1	77	Pneumonia	130	10	39	6 ± 0.3[b]
						39 ± 1.2[b]
Alzheimer 2	76	Pneumonia	120	8.3	24	97 ± 0.16[b]

[a]PNMT activity was measured in dialyzed supernatant of locus coeruleus tissue obtained at autopsy according to methods previously described (see text). Each mean (± SE) is derived from two replicate assays.

[b]$p < 0.005$ when average PNMT in Alzheimer cases (47.3 ± 21.7 pmole/hr/g) is compared to controls (293.3 ± 22.2).

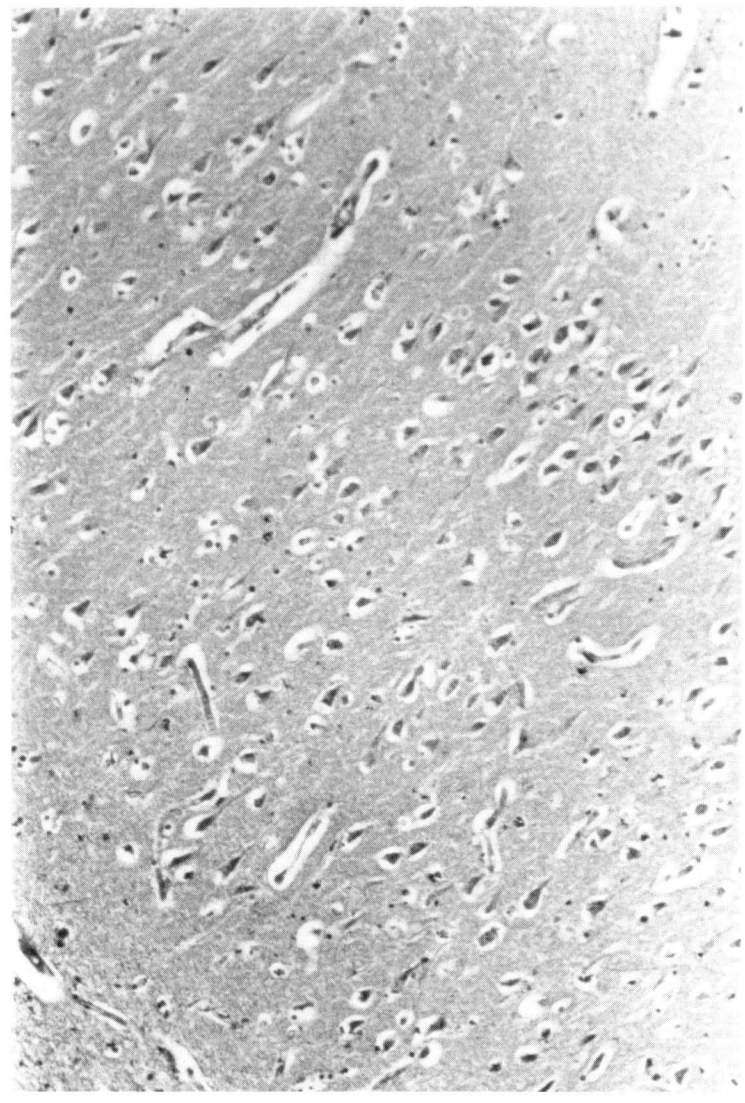

FIG 3(A). Hippocampal neurons from control case #6 (A) and Alzheimer case #2 (B). Comparable sections through the hippocampus from a control and an Alzheimer patient were stained with Bielschowsky silver stain. The large arrow indicates a senile plaque; the small arrow points to one of many neurofibrillary tangles. Magnification 31.25x.

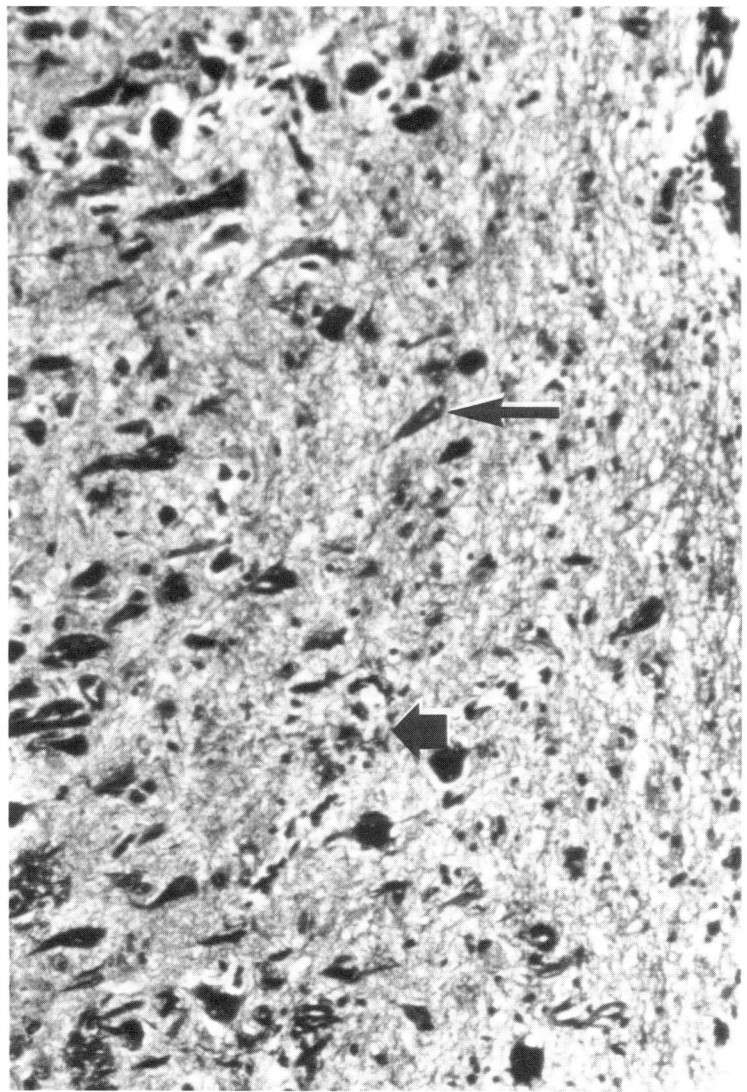

FIG. 3(B). See Fig. 3(A) legend.

Several postmortem factors which might affect PNMT were also examined (Table 3). The cause of death, length of interval from death to refrigeration (57-220 min), length of interval from death to autopsy (13.2-22.6 hr), and length of time from autopsy to assay during which tissue was frozen at -70° C (2-137 days), were either similar or involved shorter intervals for Alzheimer cases compared to controls. We have previously noted a difference of 33 percent in PNMT between the right and left locus coeruleus in a control case. Although the degree of asymmetry was increased in Alzheimer case #1, both sides had significantly lower activity than the corresponding control tissue. Both clinical and pathological asymmetry in degenerative diseases of the central nervous system have previously been reported (16,19). The data in Tables 3 and 5 indicate that the diminished PNMT activity, found in the locus coeruleus from Alzheimer cases, is related to the disease process and not to effects of pre- or postmortem factors on PNMT.

TABLE 4. PNMT activity in various regions of human brain from a control and an Alzheimer patient[a]

Brain region	PNMT activity (pmole/hr/g)	
	Control	Alzheimer
Locus coeruleus	193.0 ± 3.30	97.0 ± 0.16[b]
Frontal (middle frontal gyrus)	47.2 ± 1.18	11.2 ± 0.8[b]
Amygdala	29.4 ± 1.45	10.4 ± 0.2[b]
Hippocampus	29.1 ± 0.44	9.3 ± 0.1[b]
Cerebellum (posterior, inferior)		44.1 ± 1.45

[a]PNMT activity was measured in dialyzed supernatant from various regions of autopsy brains from control #6 and Alzheimer #2. The PNMT assay has been described (see text). Each mean ($\pm$ SE) is derived from two replicate assays.
[b]$p < 0.01$ compared to controls.

HOW PNMT NEURONS MAY AFFECT BRAIN FUNCTION

The concentrations of epinephrine in various regions of human brain are only 4-20 percent those of norepinephrine (2,45). Both compounds are neurotransmitters (60) which can affect brain functions directly. Our results (Table 1, Fig. 1) indicate that epinephrine neurons like norepinephrine neurons project widely throughout the brain and appear to innervate brain blood vessels as well as other neurons. Although both types of neurons have similarities, their effects on brain function may differ. There is evidence that epinephrine and norepinephrine may affect different subpopulations of neurons (64). In addition, epinephrine has a higher affinity than norepinephrine for alpha-2 and beta-2 receptor subtypes (6,15,18,64,66), including receptors in the human cortex (48).

One mechanism by which epinephrine could affect brain function is through effects on cerebral blood vessels, both directly and secondary to its effect on the locus coeruleus neurons known to innervate intracerebral microvessels (20,61). Receptors on these microvessels regulate blood flow as well as the blood-brain barrier (1,27,33,54). Stimulation of the locus coeruleus norepinephrine neurons decreases cerebral blood flow, increases the blood-brain barrier permeability to water and decreases glucose uptake (1,54). These functions of cerebral blood vessels may also be affected by epinephrine neurons.

A second mechanism by which PNMT neurons could affect brain function is through the direct effect of epinephrine on other neurons. In addition to the well-known subcortical projections of PNMT neurons to brainstem, diencephalon and basal ganglia (35,37,47), our results show a wider distribution of PNMT to the cortex including the frontal, parietal, and occipital regions as well as hippocampus and amygdala. The subcortical projections of the C-1 and C-2 PNMT neurons have been postulated to play a role in several brain functions including regulation of food and water intake (22), body temperature (38), blood pressure (66), and sleep (23) (Table 6). The latter two functions have been attributed to inhibitory synapses of epinephrine on the locus coeruleus neurons (22,23,66). In addition to these autonomic functions, higher cortical functions of mood and memory (22,25,26,40,41) may be influenced by epinephrine. Consolidation of memory during the storage process has been localized to the amygdala and hippocampus (41,46). Epinephrine, injected subcutaneously as well as intraventricularly in rats, modulates the memory storage process (40). The subcutaneous dose of epinephrine required to affect memory storage was 500 times that needed to get a similar response with intraventricular catecholamine (40). This suggests that the effect of epinephrine on memory storage could be mediated by very small amounts of epinephrine which may cross the blood-brain barrier. Our results showing the presence of PNMT, the enzyme marker for epinephrine in human amygdala and hippocampus (Table 1), are compatible with the hypothesis that small amounts of epinephrine may contribute to memory storage processing. The Alzheimer's disease patients were noted to have deficits in several of the functions (Table 5) which have been attributed to the presence of epinephrine including alterations in sleep, blood pressure, mood, and memory (Table 6).

TABLE 5. Clinical characteristics of control and Alzheimer patients

Characteristic	Control 1	Control 2	Control 3	Control 4	Control 5	Control 6	Alzheimer 1	Alzheimer 2
Age (years)	68	63	40	58	69	79	77	76
Sex	M	M	M	M	M	M	M	F
Mental status	Normal	Normal	Normal	Normal	Normal	Disorientation with fluctuating deficits in memory, attention, spatial orientation	Disoriented with deficits in memory, attention, spatial orientation abstraction calculation, visual perception, sleep, gait apraxia	Disoriented, mute, incontinent
Duration of AD (years)							4	11

TABLE 5 (continued). Clinical characteristics of control and Alzheimer patients

Characteristic	Control 1	Control 2	Control 3	Control 4	Control 5	Control 6	Alzheimer 1	Alzheimer 2
Diagnoses[a]	PN,H, TB,PNX	ETOH, CIR, ASC, PhCa, PN,CA, RF	L Ca,A PN	L Ca, Br Mets SCZ, GIH,A, PE	COPD, CORP, CHF, SLA, ETOH, GIH,A	HTN,ATH,ASHD, CHF,RF,COPD,DU, GIH,ST,OBS	AD,HTN,ADOM, ATH,ASHD,RF, GL,PN,SZ	AD, PN, SZ
CNS, receptor[b] medications at time of death	Mp, Digox, Theo	Lt, Cm, Theo	Hy, Mor	Fl, Trihex, Cm, Dex	Digox, Theo	Prazocin, Cimetidine	Timolol Pilocarpine	Digoxin
Length of Coma	0.5 hr	0.5 hr	4.5 hr	6.75 hr	0.8 hr	4 days	1 day	2 days

[a]Abbreviations: A, anemia; AD, Alzheimer's disease; ADOM, diabetes mellitus; ASC, ascites; ASHD, arteriosclerotic heart disease; ATH, generalized atherosclerosis; Br Mets, brain metastasis; CA, cardiac arrest; CHF, congestive heart failure; CIR, cirrhosis; CNS, central nervous system; COPD, chronic obstructive pulmonary disease; CORP, cor pulmonale; DU, duodenal ulcer; ETOH, ethanol abuse; GIH, gastrointestinal hemorrhage; GL, glaucoma; H, hypoxia; HTN, hypertension; L Ca, lung cancer; OBS, organic brain syndrome; Ph Ca, pharyngeal cancer; PE, pulmonary emboli; PN, pneumonia, PNX, pneumonectomy; RF, renal failure; SCZ, schizophrenia; SLA, sleep apnea; ST, senile tremor; SZ, seizures, TB, tuberculosis.

[b]Abbreviations: Cm, cimetidene; Dex, dexamethasone; Digox, digoxin; Fl, fluphenazine; Hy, hydromorphone; Lt, levothyroxine; Mor, morphine; Mp, metaproterenol; Theo, theophylline; Trihex, trihexyphenidyl.

TABLE 6. Functions of brain postulated to be affected by epinephrine neurons

Sleep-wake cycle
Blood pressure
Food and water intake
Temperature regulation
Mood
Memory

MECHANISM FOR LOSS OF PNMT IN ALZHEIMER'S DISEASE

There are at least two possible mechanisms for the decrease of PNMT in the locus coeruleus and other regions from Alzheimer's disease brains. First, the deficit in this enzyme could be due to a loss of C-1 and C-2 neurons simultaneously with and by the same pathologic process which affects other classes of neurons in Alzheimer's disease (7,59,65). Alternatively, a loss of cortical and locus coeruleus neurons (7), to which PNMT neurons project, could result in transsynaptic retrograde changes in PNMT in nerve terminals (16,17,51,52). To differentiate these two mechanisms, we examined control #6 and Alzheimer #2 in more detail. The results show a significant decrease in PNMT in C-1 and C-2 projection areas including the locus coeruleus (50 percent) as well as cortical areas (65-76 percent) known to be affected by Alzheimer's disease (Table 4). There was no decrease in PNMT in the posterior cerebellum of this Alzheimer patient compared to control (Ref. 13, Tables 1 and 4); the cerebellum is an area not affected by Alzheimer's disease. Corresponding to a diminution in PNMT in the locus coeruleus and hippocampus, was a decrease in the number of postsynaptic neurons in these structures (Table 7, Fig. 1, Fig. 3). That there were decreased numbers of locus coeruleus neurons was supported by

TABLE 7. Number of neurons in the C1, C2, and locus coeruleus from a control and an Alzheimer patient[a]

Group	Cell density (number of neurons/field)		
	C-1	C-2	Locus coeruleus
Control	61 ± 3.5	35 ± 3.5	105 ± 3.3
Alzheimer	57 ± 4.6	29 ± 4.5	10 ± 1.5

[a]Sections were made through comparable areas of maximum cell density in locus coeruleus, C-1, and C-2 from control #6 and AD#2. The locus coeruleus, C-1, and C-2 tissues were stained and all neurons containing nuclei, in an area 4.8 mm^2 at a magnification of 125X, were counted. Each mean (± SE) is derived from cell counts from three sections. The sections were made at 30μ intervals.

the finding of fewer beta receptors in this area (Table 2). By contrast, there was no loss of PNMT neuronal cell bodies in the C-1 or C-2 regions (Table 7, Fig. 2), although some of these neurons appeared to be undergoing atrophy in AD #2 (Fig. 2). Decreases in catecholamine enzymes without loss of neuronal cell bodies during the retrograde reaction following axonal transsection of the locus coeruleus in rats have been noted (56). Retrograde neuronal atrophy has also been used to explain neuronal changes in the choline acetyltransferase system in the nucleus basalis in Alzheimer's disease (52). This explanation may also clarify the findings of Perry et al. (53) who reported a subgroup of Alzheimer patients with normal numbers of locus coeruleus neurons but a significant decrease in dopamine beta-hydroxylase activity in locus coeruleus projection areas in the frontal and temporal cortex. Our results indicate that similar retrograde changes may occur in C-1 and C-2 PNMT neurons in Alzheimer's disease after loss of the postsynaptic neuron. We postulate that much of the neuronal loss and consequent clinical decline in Alzheimer's disease may be due to retrograde degeneration.

FUTURE THERAPEUTIC STRATEGIES IN ALZHEIMER'S DISEASE

Our results and those of others (21) suggest that as Alzheimer's disease progresses, more transmitter systems become affected due to transsynaptic degeneration. This suggests that neurotransmitter replacement therapy may prove more difficult as the disease progresses. It will therefore be important to detect the disease early and to determine which system of neurons is affected first in Alzheimer's disease. A candidate for this role has been the cholinergic neurons in the nucleus basalis and septal regions. One therapeutic strategy would be to prevent the atrophy of the first affected neurons, in the hope that if their degeneration could be halted, the disease may not progress. In this regard, Hefti (28) has shown that intraventricular injection of nerve growth factor promotes the survival of septal cholinergic neurons in adult rats after lesions in the cholinergic septo-hippocampal pathway. This finding indicates that the nerve growth factor is able to halt the degeneration of rat forebrain cholinergic neurons after transsection of their axonal processes. However, since nerve growth factor is a large protein which does not readily cross the blood-brain barrier, there is a need to develop nerve growth factor agonists which are smaller and could get into the brain when given orally or intravenously.

Our findings of retrograde degeneration in Alzheimer's disease also imply that a buildup of the brain's own chemicals may be toxic to neurons and suggests a second therapeutic strategy. A synthetically prepared analogue of meperidine, 1-methyl-4-phenyl-1,2,4,6-tetrahydropyridine (MPTP), has recently been shown to be selectively toxic to dopaminergic neurons and to produce a Parkinson-like syndrome in drug abusers (36). These toxic effects are due not to MPTP itself but to the oxidative metabolite of MPTP (39). The toxic effects of MPTP in monkeys can be blocked by drugs which inhibit its oxidation (i.e., monamine oxidase beta inhibitors) (34). By analogy, a search for brain chemicals which could act as neuronal autotoxins (11,12) may lead to strategies to block their toxic effects on neurons.

REFERENCES

1. Abraham, W.C., Delanoy, R.L., Dunn, A.J., and Zornetzer, S.F. (1979): Brain Res., 172:387-392.
2. Adolfsson, R., Gottfries, C.G., Oreland, L., Roos, B.E., and Windblad, B. (1978): Alzheimer's Disease: Senile Dementia and Related Disorders, Vol. 7, edited by R. Katzman, R.D. Terry, and K.L. Bick, pp. 441-445. Raven Press, New York.
3. Amaducci, L., Sorbi, S., Albanese, A., and Gainotti, G. (1981): Neurology, 31:799-805.
4. Armstrong, D.M., Ross, C.A., Pickel, V.M., Joh, T.H., and Reis, D.J. (1982): J. Comp. Neurol., 212:173-187.
5. Axelrod, J. (1962): J. Biol. Chem., 237:1657-1660.
6. Bolme, P., Corrodi, H., Fuxe, K., Hokfelt, T., Lindbrink, P., and Goldstein, M. (1974): Eur. J. Pharmacol., 28:89-94.
7. Bondareff, W., Mountjoy, C.O., and Roth, M. (1982): Neurology, 32:164-168.
8. Borchardt, R.T., Vincek, W.C., and Grunewald, G.L. (1977): Anal. Biochem., 82:149-157.
9. Bowen, D.M., Smith, C.B., White, P., and Davison, A.N. (1976): Brain, 99:459-496.
10. Bulbring, E. (1949): Brit. J. Pharmacol., 4:234-240.
11. Burke, W.J., Davis, J.W., and Joh, T.H. (1983): Endocrinology, 113:1102-1110.
12. Burke, W.J., Davis, J.W., Joh, T.H., Reis, D.J., Horenstein, S., and Bhagat, B. (1978): Endocrinology, 103:358-367.
13. Burke, W.J., Hanson, D.M., and Chung, H.D. (1986): Proc. Soc. Exp. Biol. Med., (in press).
14. Bylund, D.B., and Snyder, S.H. (1976): Mol. Pharmacol., 12:568-580.
15. Bylund, D.B., and U'Prichard, D.C. (1983): Int. Rev. Neurobiol., 24:343-431.
16. Corsellis, J.A.N. (1976): In: Greenfields Neuropathology, edited by W. Blackwood and J.A.N. Corsellis, pp. 796-848. Yearbook Medical Publishers, Edinburgh.
17. Cowan, W.M. (1970): In: The Contemporary Research Methods in Neuroanatomy, edited by J.J.H. Nauta, and S.D.E. Effeson, pp. 217-251. Springer-Verlag, New York

18. Coyle, J.T., and Snyder, S.H. (1981): In: Basic Neurochemistry, edited by G.J. Siegel, R.W. Albers, B.W. Agranoff, and R. Katzman, pp. 205-218. Little, Brown and Co., Boston, Massachusetts.
19. Cummings, J.L., and Benson, D.F. (1983): Dementia: A Clinical Approach. pp. 35-69. Butterworth Publishers, Stoneham, Massachusetts.
20. Edvinsson, L. (1975): Acta Physiol. Scand. [Suppl.], 427: 1-35.
21. Francis, P.T., Palmer, A.M., Sims, N.R., Bowen, D.M., Davison, A.N., Esero, M.M., Neary, D., Snowden, J.S. and Wilcock, G.K. (1985): N. Engl. J. Med., 313:7-11.
22. Fuller, R. W. (1982): Ann. Rev. Pharmacol. Toxicol., 22: 31-55.
23. Fuxe, K., Lindbrink, P., Hokfelt, T., Bolme, P., and Goldstein, M. (1974): Acta Physiol. Scand., 91:566-567.
24. Glenner, G. G. (1984): Biochem. Biophys. Res. Commun., 120: 885-890.
25. Gold, P. E., and van Buskirk, R. (1978): Behav. Biol., 23: 509-520.
26. Gold, P. E., and van Buskirk, R. (1978): Behav. Biol., 24: 168-184.
27. Grubb, R.L., Raichle, M.E., and Eichling, J.O. (1978): Brain Res., 144:204-207.
28. Hefti, F. (1986): In: Proceedings of the International Meeting on Alzheimer's Disease and Related Neurodegenerative Disorders, edited by A. Fisher, in press. Raven Press, New York.
29. Hokfelt, T., Fuxe, K., Goldstein, M., and Johansson, O. (1973): Acta Physiol. Scand., 89:286-288.
30. Hokfelt, T., Fuxe, K., Goldstein, M., and Johansson, O. (1974): Brain Res., 66:235-251.
31. Hokfelt, T., Johansson, O., and Goldstein, M. (1984): Science, 225:1326-1334.
32. Joh, T.H., and Ross, M.E. (1983): In: Immunohistochemistry, IBRO Handbook Series, Vol. 3, edited by A. C. Cuello, pp. 131-138. John Wiley and Sons, Chichester.
33. Kobayashi, H., Memo, M., Spano, P.F., and Trabucchi, M. (1981): J. Neurochem., 36:1383-1388.
34. Kopin, I. (1985): Soc. Neurosci., 2:454.
35. Kopp, N., Denoroy, L., Renaud, B., Pujol, J.F., Tabib, A., and Tommasi, M. (1979): J. Neurol. Sci., 41:397-409.
36. Langston, J.W., Ballard, P., Tetrod, J.W. and Irwin, I. (1983): Science, 219:979-980.
37. Lew, J.Y., Matsumoto, Y., Pearson, J., Goldstein, M., Hokfelt, T., and Fuxe, K. (1977): Brain Res., 119: 199-210.
38. Liang, N.Y., Borchardt, R.T., Choi, J.C., Tessel, R. E., Grunewald, G.L. (1982): Res. Commun. Chem. Pathol. Pharmacol., 37:445-452.

39. Markey, S.P., Johannessen, J.N., and Chiven, C.C. (1984): Nature, 311:464-467.
40. McGaugh, J.L. (1983): Am. Psychol., 38:161-174.
41. McGaugh, J.L., Gold, P.E., Handwerker, M.J., Jensen, R. A., Martinez, J.L., Meligeni, J.A., and Vasquez, B.J. (1979): In: Brain Mechanisms in Memory and Learning from the Single Neuron to Man, edited by M.A.B. Brazier, pp. 151-163. Raven Press, New York.
42. McGeer, E. (1978): In: Alzheimer's Disease: Senile Dementia and Related Disorders, Vol. 7, edited by R. Katzman, R.D. Terry, and K.L. Bick, pp. 427-440. Raven Press, New York.
43. McGeer, E., and McGeer, P.L. (1976): In: Neurobiology of Aging, Vol. 3, edited by R.D. Terry, and S. Gershom, pp. 389-403. Raven Press, New York.
44. McGeer, E., McGeer, P.L., and Wada, J.A. (1971): J. Neurochem., 18:1647-1658.
45. Mefford, I., Oke, A., Keller, R., Adams, R.N., and Jonsson, G. (1978): Neurosci. Lett., 9:227-231.
46. Mishkin, M. (1978): Nature, 273:297-298.
47. Nagatsu, T., Kato, T., Numata, Y., Ikuta, K., Sano, M., Nagatsu, I., Kondo, Y., Inagaki, S., Iizuka, R., Hori, A., and Narabayashi, H. (1977): Clin. Chim. Acta, 75: 221-232.
48. Nahorski, S.R. (1978): Eur. J. Pharmacol., 51: 199-209.
49. Pearson, J., Goldstein, M., and Brandeis, L. (1979): Brain Res., 165:333-337.
50. Pearson, J., Goldstein, M., Markey, K., and Brandeis, L. (1983): Neuroscience, 8:3-32.
51. Pearson, R.C.A., Gatter, K.C., and Powell, T.P.S. (1983): Brain Res., 261:321-326.
52. Pearson, R.C.A., Sofroniew, M.V., Cuello, A.C., Powell, T.P.S., Eckenstein, E., Esiri, M.M., and Wilcock, G.K. (1983): Brain Res., 289:375-379.
53. Perry, E.K., Tomlinson, B.E., Blessed, G., Perry, R.H., Cross, A.J., and Crow, T.J. (1981): J. Neurol. Sci., 51:279-287.
54. Raichle, M.E., Hartman, B.K., Bichling, J.O., and Sharpe, L.G. (1975): Proc. Natl. Acad. Sci. USA, 72: 3726-3730.
55. Ross, C.A., Ruggiero, D.A., Joh, T.H., Park, D.H., and Reis, D.J. (1984): J. Comp. Neurol., 228:168-185.
56. Ross, R.A., Joh, T.H., and Reis, D.J. (1975): Brain Res., 92:57-72.
57. Saaverda, J.M., Coyle, J.T., and Axelrod, J. (1973): J. Neurochem., 20:743-752.
58. Saaverda, J.M., Palkovits, M., Brownstein, M.J., and Axelrod, J. (1974): Nature, 248:695-696.
59. Saper, C.B., German, D.C., and White, C.L. (1985): Neurology, 35:1089-1095.

60. Snyder, S.H., Bruns, R.F., Daly, J.W., and Innis, R.B. (1981): Fed. Proc., 40:142-146.
61. Swanson, L.W., Connelly, M.A., and Hartman, B.K. (1977): Brain Res., 136:166-173,
62. Towle, A.C., Lauder, J.M., and Joh, T.H. (1984): J. Histochem. Cytochem., 32:766-770.
63. Trocewicz, J., Oka, K., and Nagatsu, T. (1982): J. Chromatogr., 227:407-413.
64. U'Prichard, D.C., and Snyder, S.H. (1978): Eur. J. Pharmacol., 51:145-155.
65. Whitehouse, P.J., Price, D.L., Clark A.W., Coyle, J.T., and Delong, M.R. (1981): Ann. Neurol., 10:122-126.
66. Wilkening, D., Dvorkin, B., Makman, M.H., Lew, J.Y., Matsumoto, J., Baba, Y., Goldstein, M., and Fuxe, K. (1980): Brain Res., 186:133-143.

Geriatric Clinical Pharmacology,
edited by W. Gibson Wood and Randy Strong.
Raven Press, New York © 1987.

CURRENT PROGRESS IN TREATING AGE-RELATED MEMORY PROBLEMS:
A PERSPECTIVE FROM ANIMAL PRECLINICAL
AND HUMAN CLINICAL RESEARCH

Raymond T. Bartus,* ** Thomas H. Crook,***
and Reginald L. Dean*

*Department of CNS Research, Lederle Laboratories,
Medical Research Division of American Cyanamid Company,
Pearl River, New York 10965;
**New York University Medical Center,
New York, New York 10016; ***Memory Assessment Clinics, Inc.,
Bethesda, Maryland 20814.

It has become commonly recognized that the proportion and number of people over 65 years old is increasing at a rapid pace. The impact of this dramatic and unprecedented demographic shift is, in many ways, reshaping the demands placed upon medical institutions responsible for providing necessary treatment and care of society's health problems. In addition to practitioners having to be cognizant of many new complications associated with treating elderly patients with drugs, many medical researchers have refocused their attention toward understanding and ultimately treating new medical problems which were previously of only minimal importance in a younger population (126). One such problem is the gradual decline of cognitive abilities associated with advanced age. Characterized initially by a disturbance in specific types of memory ability, cognitive disturbances represent one of the primary neuropsychiatric complaints of the elderly (163). Indeed, some authorities claim that over 90 percent of all people over the age of 65 suffer measurable memory problems (171). By far, the worst incidents involve those patients afflicted with one of the age-related neurodegenerative diseases, such as Alzheimer's or Parkinson's disease, where the cognitive loss insidiously progresses to the point where the entire functional capacity of the brain is destroyed and complete institutional care is required. The tremendous psychological and financial consequences associated with these diseases (especially Alzheimer's disease) have been well-characterized in several recent volumes (44,45) and a similar detailed discussion here would be superfluous. However, it is important to note that significant age-related cognitive disturbances are hardly restricted to Alzheimer's disease. For example, it is now recognized that even normal aging is associated with a selective loss of certain mental abilities, especially those requiring memory (102). In fact, impairments in memory for recent events appear to be the price paid by members of all mammalian species who are successful in surviving into their post-reproductive, senescent years (14). In humans, normal age-related loss of memory (variously referred to as benign, senescent forgetfulness or minimal memory impairment) is considered to be one of the most consistent and dehumanizing consequences of aging (102,163).

Although the decline in memory ability in normal aging in no way approaches the more severe and broader loss of mental capacity seen in Alzheimer's disease, the effects on the individual and family can be dramatic. Performance on the job is often compromised while the quality of life can be significantly affected, particularly when the induction of secondary psychiatric symptoms such as depression occur (45,163,171). Thus, effective treatment of normal, age-related memory disturbances represents a legitimate and noble medical goal that would benefit millions (12).

The number of clinical trials attempting to identify positive pharmacological agents has markedly increased in recent years. Although a number of interesting and potentially promising approaches have emerged, no clearly effective drug has yet been discovered. Several reasons can be identified for the current lack of unqualified success, including the apparent complexity of the problem, ignorance of the underlying neurological/neurochemical variables responsible, and difficulty in controlling the clinical setting and/or accurately measuring subtle changes in clinical status. Despite these inherent problems and the limited success achieved thus far, treatment of age-related memory loss continues to represent one of the largest and most lucrative challenges facing the medical pharmaceutical industry. Although any treatment achieved within this decade would most likely neither stop the aging process, cure the victims of Alzheimer's disease, nor even completely reverse the primary symptoms, significant relief of the cognitive deficit would greatly increase the quality of life of all involved and markedly reduce the financial and emotional consequences associated with it. This chapter will review the progress that has been made in this area and provide a state-of-the-art perspective as to what is known regarding various treatment approaches, both in terms of human clinical tests, as well as effects in one representative animal model--that using aging nonhuman primates (10,17).

PROBABLE CAUSES OF GERIATRIC MEMORY LOSS

Before reviewing various treatment approaches, a brief discussion of current thinking about the causes of the memory loss might be useful. There are a number of factors that can be identified which contribute to the loss of memory and related functions in elderly persons (47,123). Although nonorganic variables involving lifestyle and emotional state of mind certainly contribute to changes in intellectual capacity in old age (5), there is no longer any question that dysfunctions in central nervous system (CNS) activity most often contribute significantly (127).

For years, a combination of circumstantial evidence and intuitive logic contributed to the classical view that mental decline was caused by hardening of the arterial system to the brain. However, it is now commonly accepted that a reduction in blood supply to the brain, per se, is not a primary factor responsible for reduced neural function in elderly patients (32,154). Even in the cases of multi-infarct dementia, where a vascular involvement has been identified, it is clear that the primary cause of the memory loss and other behavioral symptoms stems from the resultant neurological destruction, and not a continued interruption in blood supply (81,156). Evidence for a similar neurological and/or neurochemical explanation of the memory loss in normal aging has also accumulated during the last several years (8,34,72,73,91,142).

Although we are still far from fully understanding how the brain functions to allow us to learn and remember, let alone what goes wrong in old age and dementia, some encouraging lines of evidence have developed. Of the many neurochemical and histological changes that have been characterized in brain tissue from aged humans and animals, the two which receive the greatest support for a relationship to the age-related cognitive deficits are impaired neuronal metabolic capacity and reduced cholinergic function (19,25,42,48). More recently, the involvement of other neurotransmitter systems and combinations or imbalances of neurotransmitter systems has been proposed (see 22 for review). Although the problem will most certainly prove to be more complex than any of these explanations can presently offer, they do provide a sufficient empirical foundation to direct the development of animal models, screening schemes, and chemical synthesis for a discovery program aimed at successfully satisfying contemporary medical expectations. Sufficient evidence is also accumulating to develop a rationale for conducting clinical trials in humans.

From a somewhat different perspective, laboratory studies have recently demonstrated that memory loss occurs with advanced age in many mammals including numerous species of mice (21,55,105,151), rats (76,108), and monkeys (10,15,54,114,118). This impairment is conceptually and operationally similar to that suffered, to varying degrees, by advanced aged and early demented humans (69). Cross-species similarity supports the idea that the memory loss associated with advanced age and dementia share similar biological underpinnings, and that aged animals might be useful as model systems for studying age-associated memory loss and potential treatment approaches (10,20,25). Recent studies with reference drugs suggest that pharmacological data from logically-derived animal models can be used to verify weak clinical observations as well as provide a rationale to help direct future clinical trials in the area of geriatric psychopharmacology (14,17,20,25). Thus, the use of aged animals and appropriate behavioral paradigms to measure loss of memory provides an additional empirical tool for screening and developing drugs intended to reduce the memory losses associated with old age and dementia.

We are only beginning to unravel the variables responsible for the loss of cognitive capacity in old age or dementia (157). However, a number of empirical findings can be applied to help toward the development of drugs to be used in clinical trials.

CURRENT PHARMACOLOGICAL APPROACHES FOR AGE-RELATED COGNITIVE DISTURBANCES

Despite the magnitude of the problem and the marked concern of patients and medical authorities, there exist no commonly accepted means of effectively treating the memory loss associated with old age or dementia at present. Several different approaches have been tried in the past, or are currently being used or investigated, and evidence exists that some of these alternatives may produce marginal relief of the cognitive symptoms. More importantly, information gained from some of these approaches may lead to the development of newer, truly effective therapy in the future.

Nootropics--Clinical Status

Nootropics comprise a relatively new pharmacological group of compounds intended to restore or maintain normal brain function. They are distinguished from almost all other psychotropic drugs because they are relatively devoid of the overt side effects (e.g., sedation, changes in motor activity, etc.) characteristic of other centrally acting drugs (74). In laboratory tests with animals, nootropics have been shown to preserve normal brain activity and behavior under conditions of metabolic stress and other neuronal perturbations (74,77,110,125,143). Some of the drugs in this class had been previously classified as cerebral vasodilators because an increase in blood flow to the brain was often one of the concomitant effects measured (39,40,87,93). Most authorities now believe that the changes observed in blood flow simply represent a response to increased neuronal metabolism.

Because of their pharmacological profile, nootropics are marketed widely in Europe for geriatric patients as well as for treating stroke and closed-head injuries and other conditions in which cognitive capacity is most often impaired (75). Although the definitions can be somewhat arbitrary, several different chemical entities can be logically included in this class of drugs, represented by structures as diverse as piracetam, vincamine, centrophenoxine and dihydroergotoxine (Hydergine®). Considering the several parent structures and scores of analogs, the number of drugs that can be included in the nootropic class is quite large and none enjoys a clear edge over the others in the clinic or the marketplace. Within recent years a consensus has begun to emerge that certain of these drugs may indeed induce subtle improvement in cognitive performance and global clinical status in geriatric patients.

To date, only the drug, dihydroergotoxine, has Food and Drug Administration (FDA) approval for treating cognitive-related problems of the elderly. Dihydroergotoxine consists of a mixture of four different ergot alkaloids in their dihydrogenated forms (85). Although it is known to have vasodilator effects, many investigators now believe its primary mechanism of action involves either direct or indirect effects on neurotransmission and/or enhancement of cerebral metabolic efficiency (64,87,93,103,110,143). Dihydroergotoxine gained FDA approval in 1973 under now-obsolete guidelines for efficacy established by the Federal Food, Drug and Cosmetics Act of 1962. Its efficacy remains controversial to this day, and most objective evaluations rate it as only marginally active, at best (71,90,92,112,116).

Many clinical reports of mild improvement under dihydroergotoxine have been published (101; reviewed in 71 and 116) but these most often involve effects on a broad range of subjective symptoms, typically assessed through patient reports and clinical observation (92,116). Rather than directly affecting cognitive ability, it appears that the drug subtly improves global clinical status through a mild activating or mood elevating effect (116,168,170). Further, the clinical meaning of the rather modest changes in subjective rating scales has been questioned recently (33,83,106,139,141,169). Despite these problems and the fact that surveys indicate that most practicing physicians believe dihydroergotoxine to be ineffective, its sales in 1983 were $35 million in the United States and over $260 million internationally.

Among the other nootropics, piracetam has clearly attracted the greatest investigational attention in the United States, both in terms of direct interest in the compound itself, and in the chemical synthesis of chemically related analogs by other drug companies. Piracetam has effects on brain energy metabolism, facilitates performance on measures of learning and retention in brain lesioned and aged rats, and protects against hypoxia-induced memory impairment in animals (74,125). Controlled studies with piracetam in Alzheimer's disease and other age-related cognitive disorders to date have been equivocal (2,35,80,104,109,119,128,150). Interestingly, some of the more impressive results of piracetam include reducing the symptoms of acute alcohol withdrawal (75), improving recovery from closed head injuries (1,82), and in treating dyslexic children (146,147,160,166). Recently, a combination treatment of piracetam plus lecithin was found to be more effective than either drug alone in facilitating memory in aged rats (23). Preliminary analysis of clinical studies in five different geriatric centers suggest that some patients with Alzheimer's disease may respond positively to this treatment (67,70,79,144,149). However, any consistently positive effects are likely to be quite subtle.

Several close analogs of piracetam have been synthesized and developed by other pharmaceutical companies. Some of these piracetam analogs have now been tested in Alzheimer patients, including several double-blind, multicenter studies. Any conclusion as to whether these drugs represent significant improvement over the extremely modest effects of piracetam would be premature and must await the outcome of peer review and publication of these studies.

Nootropics--Effects in Aged Monkeys

Because the very efficacy of nootropics is still open to question, representative drugs were administered to aged monkeys using a model procedure sensitive to the type of memory loss suffered by senescent human and early Alzheimer patients. In the first study, piracetam, vincamine, and dihydroergotoxine were administered to aged Rhesus monkeys (over 18 years) chronically in a counter-balanced manner for a minimum of nine consecutive days (p.o.,b.i.d.) (13). A washout period of a minimum of one week occurred between drugs. The results demonstrated that all three drugs produced some improvement in performance in the aged monkeys. Not all monkeys demonstrated the same qualitative response, i.e., some exhibited clear improvement, others showed no change, and still a few isolated cases showed mild impairments compared to the nondrug control scores. These effects agree with the general findings of many clinical trials described earlier.

More recently, we compared the effects of chronic administration of piracetam and centrophenoxine in aged Cebus monkeys (over 18 years) and very similar effects were obtained (13). Again, certain monkeys exhibited reliable increases in performance whereas others showed no apparent improvement. The fact that reliable positive effects were obtained with certain memory-impaired subjects but not others, provides an objective reason to be encouraged that the nonhuman primate may be useful

for determining why some elderly patients respond favorably to
some of these agents while others do not. One possibility is
that the memory loss seen in aging is the result of a complex,
multifaceted etiology and thus, only a subpopulation of
geriatric patients will respond to this type of treatment.
Further characterization of this subpopulation to determine
possible differences in the behavioral and neurochemical
deficits should provide invaluable information to increase our
understanding of this problem and develop effective therapy.

Cerebral Vasodilators--Clinical Status

As discussed in the section on "Causes of Geriatric Memory
Loss," evidence for a cerebral-vascular role in the disorder
was primarily circumstantial, and the logic intuitive. After
enjoying years of popularity, the concept no longer is held in
high regard by leading authorities. Historically, it grew out
of the hypothesis that dementia results from cerebral
arteriosclerosis and reduced blood flow (6,39). More recently,
it has been argued that even in those minority cases where a
vascular etiology is implicated, vasodilator therapy could
likely reduce needed blood flow to ischemic or arteriosclerotic
areas (by preferentially dilating vessels in healthier, more
responsive brain regions); thus, exacerbating the
neurobehavioral symptoms (135). A number of cerebral
vasodilators have been carefully studied in geriatric clinics
(6,39,40,93,169), and very little evidence for continued
consideration has been generated.

Perhaps a possible exception to this may be papaverine for
which evidence of positive (albeit controversial) effects have
been reported (93,169). However, in four separate studies
which directly compared papaverine to dihydroergotoxine,
dihydroergotoxine was found consistently to be more effective
(26,63,124,138). Although it was once assumed that the
possible beneficial effects of papaverine were related to its
vasodilator activity (117), lack of similar efficacy with many
other vasodilators has questioned this interpretation. Its
abilities to block dopamine receptors (61,145) and to inhibit
phosphodiesterase (120,131) have been suggested recently as
possible mechanisms of action.

There presently exists little theoretical or empirical
support for the use of vasodilators in treating age-related
cognitive impairments. It should be recognized that despite
this fact, some unenlightened physicians continue to prescribe
vasodilators for this purpose.

Anticoagulants (and Rheologic Agents)--Clinical Status

A variation on the theme that vascular problems contribute
to the cognitive impairments of age and dementia postulates
that changes in red blood cells may reduce oxygen supply to the

brain. Specifically, blood sludging, which involves the intravascular adhesion or clumping of red blood cells, is known to occur as a natural consequence of disease or physical trauma (100). It has been suggested that sludged blood also increases with age and dementia (99), and may impair brain function through a number of factors including decreased oxygen availability to the brain, as well as alterations in the blood-brain barrier (27,46). Although preliminary and controversial clinical studies in the 1970's suggested that sludged blood may play an important role in the etiology of senility (161,162), no confirmation of these findings has been published (see 115).

Although not specifically an anticoagulant, pentoxifylline (Trental®) has been shown to improve blood flow in regions of arterial/venous restriction by lowering blood viscosity and improving red cell flexibility (88,94,121,122). In fact, pentoxifylline has recently been approved by the FDA for the treatment of intermittent claudication (4), suffered by 2 to 4 million people in the United States. People afflicted with intermittent claudication have difficulty walking due to numbness, cramping and pain in the leg. The condition results from inadequate blood flow to the extremities. In a number of geriatric clinics, pentoxifylline is currently being tested for multi-infarct dementia, stroke, and Alzheimer's disease.

Anticoagulants--Data from Aged Monkeys

Relatively little animal data are available regarding the relationship between age, blood sludging, and behavioral changes. Malcolm et al. (113) reported an impairment in performance on a delayed discrimination task with chemically induced sludged blood in healthy adult rats. Since an impairment was found only under the delayed condition, and not under the immediate discrimination condition, their data suggested that sludged blood may preferentially impair recent memory and therefore could conceivably contribute to memory loss that occurs in aged and demented patients. We attempted to evaluate this possibility in greater detail to determine the empirical validity of this approach.

In this study, two interrelated, logical approaches were used (115). In the first, sludged blood was artificially (chemically) induced in younger rats, and their behavior was evaluated for effects on memory performance. The rationale of this approach was that if sludged blood is primarily responsible for age-related decline in recent memory, then induced sludged blood in young, healthy animals should result in behavioral deficits qualitatively similar to those observed in old age. The second approach involved evaluating the blood from young and aged monkeys to determine whether those monkeys with severe memory impairments have increased sludged blood.

In the first procedure, blood sludging was induced in young rats (3 months old) with intravenous injections of high molecular weight dextran. Previous studies revealed that a 300 mg/kg dose produced a tenfold increase in the erythrocyte sedimentation rate, a quantitative measure of the degree of blood sludging. The performance of the dextran-treated rats on a delayed, spatial alternation task was measured at various delay intervals (15-120 seconds) and compared to the nondextran control scores. The data demonstrated that the accuracy of performance on the delayed alternation procedure was not reduced after the dextran treatment. The only obvious behavioral effect of dextran was a significant drop in the number of trials completed during the session. Further studies revealed that dextran suppressed general responding in a dose-dependent manner without significantly impairing accuracy (115).

In the second procedure, the blood from young (5-8 years) and aged (18-24 years) Rhesus monkeys that differed significantly in their recent memory ability, was examined to compare the degree of blood sludging in each group and determine whether sludging was correlated with performance on our memory task. Although the aged animals showed a trend toward a higher erythrocyte sedimentation rate, no statistically significant differences were found between the two age groups, and considerable overlap existed between age groups for the degree of sludging. Because a similar overlap does not exist in the memory ability of the two age groups, blood sludging does not appear to be a prominent or consistent feature in the physiological changes seen with aging in Rhesus monkeys and does not seem to be well-correlated with the memory deficits observed on this task. While claims of the clinical efficacy of anticoagulant therapy in some senile patients require further replication and study to explain such effects, our results offer no support for increased blood sludging as an adequate explanation for age-related impairments in memory and cannot be justified to support further attempts to treat these impairments with anticoagulation therapy.

Central Nervous System Stimulants--Clinical Status

Historically, one of the more persistent approaches applied toward the therapeutic management of the aged has been centrally acting neural stimulants (111). It had been assumed by clinicians that through their euphoric, mood-lifting, or general energizing effects, CNS stimulants might counteract age-related problems involving fatigue, inattention, learning and memory difficulties, motivation, depression, motor dysfunctions, etc. (107). Despite this early popularity, the efficacy of such treatment has never been satisfactorily established (for review, see 7,43,95). The majority of human clinical literature indicates that CNS stimulants generally do not improve, and very often impair, performance of tasks involving recent memory (7,43,134).

Central Nervous System Stimulants--Effects in Aged Monkeys

In an effort to help clarify this issue and provide a basis for direct comparison of the effects of various CNS stimulants with other pharmacological agents, the four different CNS stimulants (methylphenidate, magnesium pemoline, pentylenetetrazole/niacin mixture, and caffeine) were compared over a range of doses for their ability to enhance recent memory performance in impaired, aged (19-23 years) and unimpaired Rhesus monkeys 5 to 6 years of age (11). The first three drugs were selected because of the contemporary claims of possible efficacy in geriatric behavioral disorders while caffeine was tested to control for possible nonspecific CNS stimulant effects of the drugs.

This comparison demonstrated that none of the four CNS stimulants significantly improved (but often impaired) performance in this memory task. Methylphenidate and caffeine impaired the performance of both age groups even at relatively low doses. In contrast, magnesium pemoline produced fewer adverse effects and even demonstrated some improvement in performance though not quite statistically significant ($p < .06$). The pentylenetetrazole/niacin mixture resulted in different effects in the two age groups. The young group's responses to this drug followed a typical, progressive dose-response function with a suggestion of improvement (but not significant, $p > .05$) at the lowest dose and a significant impairment at the highest dose. The aged monkeys responded differently to this drug mixture following an inverted U-shaped function. Significant impairment was seen at the lowest dose, relatively little change in performance at the next two higher doses, and finally significant impairment at the highest dose.

These data are consistent with the majority of human clinical literature which indicates that CNS stimulants generally do not improve and very often impair performance of tasks involving recent memory (7,43,134). CNS stimulants also have numerous adverse side effects such as cardiac stimulation, increased irritability, decreased appetite, and rapid development of tolerance. To the degree to which conclusions from animal research can be generalized to humans, these data offer little support for the idea that general CNS stimulation represents an effective approach for the treatment of cognitive impairments that accompany old age.

Neuropeptides and Other Endogenous Substances--Clinical Status

In recent years, evidence has accumulated that neuropeptides of hypothalamic and pituitary origin may influence behavior, independent of their neuroendocrine effects (reviewed in

56,137). These extra-endocrine effects appear to occur by directly influencing the CNS and are long-lasting despite the short half-lives of the neuropeptides (98).

One current hypothesis is that neuropeptides stimulate their target cells in the brain through receptor-coupled second messenger systems (165). The action of the second messenger system (i.e., cAMP, cGMP, calmodulin) is to modulate protein kinase activity which governs the production and degradation of phosphoproteins. These phosphoproteins then specify the effector cell's response. Thus, it is believed neuropeptides function either as neurotransmitters or modulators of neurotransmitters, resulting in a long-lasting neurochemical change (i.e., modulation of nucleic acids and proteins) which is reflected in subsequent behavior.

Behaviorally, it has been demonstrated repeatedly that many neuropeptides, particularly vasopressin and adrenocorticotropin hormone (ACTH), affect measures of attention, anxiety, and learning and memory in several mammalian species (reviewed in 137,153,158). Interestingly, these are some of the same behaviors which have been commonly reported in the geriatric literature to be significantly altered with age (163). Unfortunately, most studies using patients with cognitive impairments (due to advanced age, dementia, stroke, or head injuries) have generally failed to show significant improvement with available neuropeptides on tasks intended to measure memory or related cognitive skills (reviewed in 68,152). It appears that the principal effects of the ACTH peptides are on mood and attention rather than on learning and memory (132). In this regard, the effect of these peptides may resemble those seen with dihydroergotoxine and similar drugs. Similarly, vasopressin peptides appear to produce nonspecific CNS stimulation rather than direct improvement of memory or other cognitive functions impaired in Alzheimer's disease (66). Whatever the clinical response might be, the magnitude of change observed in studies with Alzheimer patients using currently available peptides has been quite modest or negative (68,152).

A study by Reisberg et al. (136) recently generated considerable interest by suggesting that the narcotic antagonist, naloxone, may be of clinical value in treating Alzheimer's disease. However, other evidence questions the utility of the drug (38,159) and, at present, several well-controlled studies to determine whether the drug is clinically effective in Alzheimer's disease have reported negative results (28,129,133). Evidence from animal studies suggest that like the ACTH and vasopressin peptides, the primary effects of the drug may be on attentional processes rather than learning and memory (3).

Neuropeptides--Effects on Aged Monkeys

To further evaluate the effects of these and other neuropeptides on age-related memory impairments under controlled laboratory conditions, $ACTH_{4-10}$, lysine vasopressin, arginine vasopressin, oxytocin, and somatostatin were compared in our aged primate model (16). $ACTH_{4-10}$, the behaviorally active amino acid sequence of the anterior pituitary ACTH, is devoid of endocrine effects and has been shown to influence learning and memory. Vasopressin, also known as antidiuretic hormone, has two forms (56). One is lysine vasopressin which is unique to pigs and is the form used in several of the earlier clinical trials involving memory. The other is arginine vasopressin and is common to most mammals including human and nonhuman primates. Oxytocin, which like vasopressin is secreted from the posterior pituitary, has been shown to impair memory in young rats and humans (29,30,65). Finally, somatostatin, a hypothalamic hormone which inhibits the release of growth hormone, has been observed to decrease significantly in the brains of Alzheimer patients (49,50,140) and aged rodents (89).

None of the neuropeptides produced sufficiently consistent effects across subjects to be reflected by changes in group means. Evaluations of each individual subject against its own baseline performance revealed that all five neuropeptides produced some minimal improvement but only three of the five did so with any consistency (both forms of vasopressin and $ACTH_{4-10}$). In no case were clear, dose-response functions obtained even within individual subjects.

Arginine vasopressin produced the best overall effects with three of the five monkeys exhibiting significant improvement in performance. The same three monkeys that responded to arginine vasopressin also responded to the lysine form. Similarly, the two monkeys that failed to improve with the arginine form of vasopressin also showed no improvement with the lysine form. Although not directly compared, the effects of the arginine form appeared to be somewhat more consistent and robust than those obtained under the lysine form. It may be relevant to these results that the arginine form, but not the lysine form, of vasopressin exists naturally in human and nonhuman primates. Three of the six aged monkeys also performed better under $ACTH_{4-10}$ compared to baseline. In two of these cases, only a single dose was effective while the third improved significantly on five of six tests (two tests for each of three doses). Very little improvement in performance was observed under any dose of somatostatin or oxytocin.

These data demonstrate that reliable changes in performance on a memory task with aged primates can be achieved, suggesting that certain neuropeptides may indeed play some role in the expression or mediation of memory for recent events. The data reported here are unique in that they eliminate a popular criticism of the current literature that the data have depended

too heavily on the testing of rodents in shock-motivated
tasks. Additionally, the improvements observed in this study
involve a behavior that is naturally impaired by age and one
which has many operational similarities and some empirical
relevance to measures of recent memory in humans (13). It
might be asked as to the significance these data from aged
monkeys may have to humans. The limitations on overall
improvement seriously question the therapeutic utility of the
presently researched neuropeptides for treatment of age-related
cognitive dysfunctions. However, a consistent finding emerging
from many of the studies in aged monkeys is that certain
subpopulations of subjects exist which may respond favorably to
several potentially useful therapeutic approaches. Whether the
small improvement observed in certain aged monkeys is
indicative of a pharmacological effect that can be related to
meaningful clinical improvement in elderly humans is not
known. One optimistic possibility is that sensitive and valid
animal models, such as the one described below, will ultimately
lead to the identification of newer, neuropeptide-like
structures with more consistent and meaningful clinical effects.

Cholinomimetics--Clinical Status and Effects in Aged Monkeys

Although the relationship between age-related CNS
dysfunction and cognitive loss will prove to be complex, one
idea gaining increasing support is that a loss of CNS
cholinergic neurotransmission plays a major role in this
behavioral problem (60). This notion has come to be called the
"cholinergic hypothesis of geriatric memory"
(19,42,48,57,59,130). Over the past several years, a number of
laboratories have generated a broad range of support including
evidence from pharmacological, biochemical, and
electrophysiological studies (reviewed in 22). The cholinergic
hypothesis has also stimulated many clinical trials which have
attempted to compensate pharmacologically for the presumed
cholinergic disturbance (reviewed in 18-20,22).

These attempts can be classified into one of three
approaches: precursor therapy, anticholinesterase treatment,
and muscarinic receptor agonist treatment. Because cholinergic
precursors have a wide margin of safety and relatively loose
government regulations associated with their use, the vast
majority of these studies performed to date adopted a precursor
therapy approach. The impetus for this approach was derived
from the observation that choline availability normally limits
the rate of acetylcholine synthesis. Cohen and Wurtman (37)
and Haubrich et al. (86) independently demonstrated that acute
injections of choline chloride produced a significant,
transient effect on brain acetylcholine levels in rats and
guinea pigs. It was suggested that cholinergic function might
be therapeutically enhanced by precursor treatment (96,167).
The rationale of these precursor studies was straightforward

and conceptually similar to that used to treat other neurobehavioral disturbances with precursor loading techniques (78,167), e.g., L-dopa treatment for Parkinson's disease (41). To date, scores of clinical trials have failed to demonstrate beneficial cognitive effects with either choline or lecithin (the normal dietary source of choline) in demented or nondemented, aged patients (reviewed in 18 and 19).

By contrast, the testing of cholinergic agonists and cholinesterase inhibitors as a means of improving geriatric memory has not been as extensive as precursor therapy but has been somewhat more successful. The most popular cholinomimetic has been the anticholinesterase physostigmine. Although initial attempts to demonstrate improvement with physostigmine in geriatric patients were not successful (58,148), it is now generally accepted that physostigmine can indeed improve geriatric memory (reviewed in 18). However, as demonstrated initially in aged monkeys (9,24), the effects are quite subtle, requiring strictly controlled test conditions and special attention to large individual variations in the most effective dose. Furthermore, although these effects have been substantiated in human trials, the most consistent effects have been obtained with intravenous injections of the drug (see 18). Despite the theoretical importance of these data, their direct therapeutic relevance remains in doubt. The short half-life (53), narrow therapeutic window (51,53), variable individual dose response curve (9,18,24,36,52), and high incidence of adverse side effects (51) make physostigmine of limited value but offers clear directions for improving characteristics of new cholinergic agents.

Preliminary evidence suggests that the oral form of physostigmine may not require as much attention to individual differences in most effective doses (155). This suggestion requires confirmation (97) and there is no *a priori* reason to believe that the therapeutic effects of oral physostigmine should be more robust than those obtained with systemic injections of the drug.

The final class of cholinergics to be considered are those drugs which directly stimulate central muscarinic receptors. Preliminary studies in aged monkeys (15), as well as a report with Alzheimer patients (31,36,84) suggests direct agonists may be superior to other types of cholinergic agents in improving memory deficits. Recent reports that degeneration of cholinergic forebrain nuclei may account for the loss of choline acetyltransferase activity in Alzheimer patients provide additional impetus for studies with cholinergic agonists (42,164). If degeneration plays a major role in the cognitive symptoms of the disease, it might be assumed that the most effective treatment would be to compensate for the loss of cholinergic input to the cortex and hippocampus by stimulating the surviving postsynaptic receptors with direct muscarinic agonists. Drugs which directly stimulate postsynaptic cholinergic receptors should be more capable of improving cholinergic tone or restoring the balance of the central nervous system than drugs requiring functional, presynaptic cholinergic terminals (such as cholinergic precursors and anticholinesterases). Although there have been few studies with muscarinic agonists, the apparent advantages seen in these studies suggest that the additional clinical tests should be conducted and/or superior agonists be developed (14,17,31,36,84).

The general consensus emerging from these drug studies is that modest, but reliable improvements in human memory and related cognitive symptoms can be achieved with certain available cholinomimetics. However, in order to produce reliable effects, it is necessary to test the drug in carefully controlled clinical settings and account for relatively large, individual idiosyncrasies regarding the optimal dose (9,15,52). If effective therapy is to be achieved with cholinergic drugs, many improvements over existent cholinomimetics will have to be made. Beyond that, an approach which corrects multiple neurotransmitter deficiencies may also have to be developed (see 20 and 22 for detailed discussion).

CONCLUSIONS

Despite the growing interest and modest progress achieved in the age-related memory problems, one can safely deduce that a dramatic therapeutic advance in the near future appears unlikely. Most claims for superior activity of the newer compounds are based primarily on differences in potency and not increases in efficacy on an objective measure of memory. The need and opportunity for making a significant impact in this emerging area remains quite high.

It is important to recognize that few authoritative investigators expect any drug developed in the near future to completely reverse the cognitive dysfunction of Alzheimer's disease (20,62). However, any drug which is capable of producing a modest, but reliable improvement in a substantial proportion of the patients tested would be welcomed by all concerned parties. It is from this perspective that all current generation drugs should be developed, evaluated, and ultimately tested in clinical trials. Epidemiological and sociological studies suggest that much human suffering could be reduced and billions of dollars saved annually by patients and their families simply by increasing the intellectual capacity of Alzheimer patients to the point where self-care is possible and the need for expensive and dehumanizing institutionalization is, therefore, eliminated (126). Further, the need and opportunity to reduce natural (less severe) age-related declines (i.e., minimal memory dysfunction) should not be ignored and might even be considered a more reasonable "first goal" in this new therapeutic area (14,44).

REFERENCES

1. Aantaa, E., and Meurman, O.H. (1975): J. Int. Med. Res., 3:352-355.
2. Abuzzahab, F.S., Merwin, G.E., Zimmermann, R.L., Sherman, M.C. (1977): Pharmakopsychiatr. Neuropsychopharmakol., 10:49-56.
3. Arnsten, A.F.T. (1984): In: Alzheimer's Disease: Advances in Basic Research and Therapies, edited by R.J. Wurtman, S.H. Corkin, and J.H. Growdon, pp. 407-426. Proceedings of the Third Meeting of the International Study Group on the Treatment of Memory Disorders Associated with Aging, Zurich, Switzerland.
4. Aviado, D.M., and Porter, J.M. (1984): Pharmacotherapy, 4:297-307.
5. Avorn, J. (1983): J. Am. Geriatr. Soc., 31:137-143.
6. Ban, T.A. (1978): In: Psychopharmacology: A Generation of Progress, edited by M.A. Lipton, A. DiMascio, and K.F. Killam, pp. 1525-1533. Raven Press, New York.
7. Ban, T.A. (1980): Psychopharmacology for the Aged. Karger, New York.
8. Barbagallo-Sangiorgi G. and Exton-Smith, A.N., editors (1980): The Aging Brain: Neurological and Mental Disturbances. Plenum Press, New York.
9. Bartus, R.T. (1979a): Science, 206:1087-1089.
10. Bartus, R.T. (1979b): In: Sensory Systems and Communication in the Elderly, Vol. 10, edited by J.M. Ordy and K.R. Brizzee, pp. 85-114. Raven Press, New York.
11. Bartus, R.T. (1979c): J. Am. Geriatr. Soc., 27:289-297.
12. Bartus, R.T. (1986): In: Treatment Development Strategies for Alzheimer's Disease, edited by T. Crook, R.T. Bartus, S. Ferris, and S. Gershon, in press. Mark Powley Associates, New Canaan, Connecticut.
13. Bartus, R.T., and Dean, R.L. (1981): In: Brain Neurotransmitters and Receptors in Aging and Age-Related Disorders, Vol. 17, edited by S.J. Enna, T. Samorajski, and B. Beer, pp. 209-223. Raven Press, New York.
14. Bartus, R.T., and Dean, R.L. (1985): In: Normal Aging, Alzheimer's Disease and Senile Dementia, edited by C.G. Gottfries, pp. 231-267. University of Brussels Press, Brussels, Belgium.
15. Bartus, R.T., Dean, R.L., and Beer, B. (1980): Neurobiol. Aging, 1:145-152.
16. Bartus, R.T., Dean, R.L., and Beer, B. (1982): Neurobiol. Aging, 3:61-68.
17. Bartus, R.T., Dean, R.L., and Beer, B. (1983): Psychopharmacol. Bull., 19:168-184.
18. Bartus, R.T., Dean, R.L., and Beer, B. (1984): In: Nutrition in Gerontology, Vol. 26, edited by J.M.

Ordy, D. Harman, and R.B. Alfin-Slater, pp. 191-225. Raven Press, New York.
19. Bartus, R.T., Dean, R.L., Beer, B, and Lippa, A.S. (1982): Science, 217:408-417.
20. Bartus, R.T., Dean, R.L., and Fisher, S.K. (1986): In: Treatment Development Strategies for Alzheimer's Disease, edited by T. Crook, R.T. Bartus, S. Ferris, and S. Gershon, in press. Mark Powley Associates, New Canaan, Connecticut.
21. Bartus, R.T., Dean, R.L., Goas, J.A., and Lippa, A.S. (1980): Science, 209:301-303.
22. Bartus, R.T., Dean R.L., Pontecorvo, M.J., and Flicker, C. (1985): In: Memory Dysfunctions: An Integration of Animal and Human Research from Preclinical and Clinical Perspectives, edited by D.S. Olton, E. Gamzu, and S. Corkin, Ann. NY Acad. Sci., 444:332-358.
23. Bartus, R.T., Dean, R.L., Sherman, K.A., Friedman, E., and Beer, B. (1981): Neurobiol. Aging, 2:105-111.
24. Bartus, R.T., Fleming, D., and Johnson, H.R. (1978): J. Gerontol., 33:858-871.
25. Bartus, R.T., Flicker, C., and Dean, R.L. (1983): In: Clinical and Pre-Clinical Assessment in Geriatric Psychopharmacology, edited by T. Crook, S. Ferris, and R.T. Bartus, pp. 263-299. Mark Powley Associates, New Canaan, Connecticut.
26. Bazo, A.J. (1973): J. Am. Geriatr. Soc., 21:65-71.
27. Bicher, H.I., Bruley, D., Knisely, M.H., and Reneau, D.D. (1971): J. Physiol., 217:689-707.
28. Blass, J.P., Reding M.J., Drachman, D., Mitchell, A., Glosser, G., Katzman, R., Thal, L.J., Grenell, S., Spar, J.E., Larue, A., and Liston, E. (1983): N. Engl. J. Med., 309:556.
29. Bohus, B., Kovacs, G.L., and DeWied, D. (1978): Brain Res., 157:414-417.
30. Bohus, B., Urban, I., van Wimersma Greidanus, T.B., and DeWied, D. (1977): Neuropharmacology, 12:239-247.
31. Caine, E.D. (1980): N. Engl. J. Med., 303:585-586.
32. Caplan, L.R. (1979): In: Drug Therapy Reviews, Vol. 2, edited by R.R. Miller and D.J. Greenblatt, pp. 305-317, Elsevier, New York.
33. Castleden, C.M. (1984): J. R. Coll. Physicians Lond., 18:28-31.
34. Cervos-Navarro, J., and Sarkander, H.I., editors (1983): Brain Aging: Neuropathology and Neuropharmacology, Vol. 21. Raven Press, New York.
35. Chouinard, G., Annable, L., Ross-Chouinard, A., Olivier, M., Fontaine, F. (1983): Psychopharmacology, 81:100-106.
36. Christie, J.E., Shering, A., Ferguson, J., and Glen, A.I.M. (1981): Br. J. Psychiatry, 138:46-50.

37. Cohen, E.L., and Wurtman, R.J. (1975): *Life Sci.*, 16:1095-1102.
38. Cohen, R.M., Cohen, M.R., Weingartner, H., Pickar, D., and Murphy, D.L. (1983): *Psychiatr. Res.*, 8:127-136.
39. Cook, P., and James, I. (1981a): *N. Engl. J. Med.*, 305:1508-1513.
40. Cook, P., and James, I. (1981b): *N. Engl. J. Med.*, 305:1560-1564.
41. Cotzins, G.C., VanWoert, M.H., and Schiffer, L.M. (1967): *N. Engl. J. Med.*, 276:374-379.
42. Coyle, J.T., Price, D.L., and DeLong, M.R. (1983): *Science*, 219:1184-1190.
43. Crook, T. (1979): *J. Am. Geriatr. Soc.*, 27:476-477.
44. Crook, T., Bartus, R.T., Ferris, S., and Gershon, S. editors (1986): *Treatment Development Strategies for Alzheimer's Disease*, in press. Mark Powley Associates, New Canaan, Connecticut.
45. Crook, T., Ferris, S., and Bartus, R.T. editors (1983): *Clinical and Pre-Clinical Assessment in Geriatric Psychopharmacology*. Mark Powley Associates, New Canaan, Connecticut.
46. Cullen, C.F., and Swank, R.L. (1954): *Circulation*, 9:335-346.
47. Cummings, J., Benson, D.F., and LoVerme, S. (1980): *JAMA*, 243:2434-2439.
48. Davies, P. (1981): In: *Strategies for the Development of an Effective Treatment for Senile Dementia*, edited by T. Crook, and R.S. Gershon, pp. 19-32. Mark Powley Associates, New Canaan, Connecticut.
49. Davies, P., Katzman, R., and Terry, R.D. (1980): *Nature*, 228:279-280.
50. Davies, P., and Terry, R.D. (1981): *Neurobiol. Aging*, 2:9-14.
51. Davis, K.L., Hollister, L.E., Overall, J., Johnson, A., and Train, K. (1976): *Psychopharmacology* (Berlin), 51:23-27.
52. Davis, K.L., Mohs, R.C., and Tinklenberg, J.R. (1979): *N. Engl. J. Med.*, 301:946.
53. Davis, K.L., Mohs, R.C., Tinklenberg, J.R., Pfefferbaum, A., Hollister, L.E., and Kopell, B.S. (1978): *Science*, 20:272-274.
54. Davis, R.T. (1978): *Exp. Gerontol.*, 13:237-250.
55. Dean, R.L., Scozzafava, J., Goas, J.A., Regan, B., Beer, B., and Bartus, R.T. (1981): *Exp. Aging Res.*, 7:427-451.
56. DeWied, D. (1980): *Proc. R. Soc. Lond. (Biol)*, 210:183-195.
57. Drachman, D.A. (1977): *Neurology (Minneap.)*, 27:783-790
58. Drachman, D.A. (1978): In: *Psychopharmacology: A Generation of Progress*, edited by M.A. Lipton, A. DiMascio, and K.F. Killam, pp. 651-662. Raven Press, New York.

59. Drachman, D.A. (1983): In: Aging of the Brain, Vol. 22, edited by D. Samuel, S. Algeri, S. Gershon, V.E. Grimm, and G. Toffano, pp. 19-31. Raven Press, New York.
60. Drachman, D.A., and Leavitt, J. (1974): Arch. Neurol., 30:113-121.
61. Duvoisin, R.C. (1975): JAMA, 231:845.
62. Editorial (1984): Lancet ii:1313-1314.
63. Einspruch, B.C. (1976): Dis. Nervous System, 37:439-442.
64. Emmenegger, H., and Meier-Ruge, W. (1968): Pharmacology, 1:65-78.
65. Ferrier, B.M., Kennett, D.J., and Devlin, M.C. (1980): Life Sci., 27:2311-2317.
66. Ferris, S.H. (1983): In: Alzheimer's Disease, edited by B. Reisberg, pp. 369-373. The Free Press, New York.
67. Ferris, S.H., Reisberg, B., Friedman, E., Schneck, M.K., Sherman, K.A., Mir, P., and Bartus, R.T. (1982): Psychopharm. Bull., 18:94-98.
68. Ferris, S.H., Reisberg, B., and Gershon, S. (1980): In: Aging in the 1980's: Psychological Issues, edited by L.W. Poon, pp. 212-220. American Psychological Association, Washington, D.C.
69. Flicker, C., Ferris, S.H., Bartus, R.T., and Crook, T. (1984): Neurobiol. Aging, 5:275-282.
70. Friedman, E., Sherman, K.A., Ferris, S.H., Reisberg, B., Bartus, R.T., and Schneck, M.K. (1981): N. Engl. J. Med., 304:1490-1491.
71. Gaitz, C.M., and Hartford, J.T. (1980): In: Ergot Compounds and Brain Function: Neuroendocrine and Neuropsychiatric Aspects, edited by M. Goldstein, pp. 349-356. Raven Press, New York.
72. Giacobini, E., Filogano, G., and Vernadakis, A., editors (1982): The Aging Brain: Cellular and Molecular Mechanisms of Aging in the Nervous System, Vol. 20. Raven Press, New York.
73. Gispen, W.H., and Traber, J., editors (1982): Aging of the Brain. Proceedings of the First International Tropon Symposium on Brain Aging, Elsevier, New York.
74. Giurgea, C.E. (1976): Curr. Dev. Psychopharmacol., 3:223-273.
75. Giurgea, C.E. (1981): Fundamentals to the Pharmacology of the Mind. Thomas Publishers: Springfield, Illinois.
76. Gold, P.E., and McGaugh, J.L. (1975): In: Advances in Behavioral Biology: Neurobiology of Aging. Vol. 16, edited by J.M. Ordy, and K.R. Brizzee, pp. 145-158. Plenum Press, New York.
77. Gouret, C., and Raynard, G. (1976): J. Pharmacol. (Paris), 7:161-175.
78. Growdon, J.H. (1979): In: Nutrition and the Brain, Disorders of Eating: Nutrients in Treatment of Brain Diseases, Vol. 3, edited by R.J. Wurtman, and J.J. Wurtman, pp. 177-181. Raven Press, New York.

79. Growdon, J., Corkin, S., and Huff, F.J. (1984): In: Alzheimer's Disease: Advances in Basic Research and Therapies, edited by R.J. Wurtman, S. Corkin, and J.H. Growdon, pp. 375-390. Proceedings of the Third Meeting of the International Study Group on the Treatment of Memory Disorders Associated with Aging, Zurich, Switzerland.
80. Gustafson, L., Reisberg, J., Johanson, M., Fransson, M., and Maximillian, V.A. (1978): Psychopharmacology, 56:115-117.
81. Hachinski, V.C., Lassen, N.A., and Marshall, J. (1974): Lancet ii:207-210.
82. Hakkarainen, H., and Hakamies, L. (1978): Eur. Neurol., 17:50-55.
83. Hamilton, M. (1982): Gerontology, 28(suppl. 2):42-48.
84. Harbaugh, R.E., Roberts, D.W., Coombs, D.W. Saunders, R.L., and Reeder, T.M. (1984): Neurosurgery, 15:514-518.
85. Hartmann, V., Rodiger, M., Ableidinger, W., and Bethke, H. (1978): J. Pharm. Sci., 67:98-103.
86. Haubrich, D.R., Wang, P.F.L., Clody, D.E., and Wedeking, P.W. (1975): Life Sci., 17:975-980.
87. Hauth, H., and Richardson, B.P. (1977): In: Annual Reports in Medicinal Chemistry, Vol. 12, edited by F.H. Clarke, pp. 49-59. Academic Press, New York.
88. Heidrich, H., Schlichting, K., and Ott, M. (1976): IRCS Medical Science, 4:368.
89. Hoffman, G.E., and Sladek, J.R. (1980): Neurobiol. Aging, 1:27-38.
90. Hollister, L.E., and Yesavage, J. (1984): Ann. Intern. Med., 100:894-898.
91. Hoyer, S., editor (1982): The Aging Brain, Springer-Verlag, New York.
92. Hughes, J.J., Williams, J.G., and Currier, R.D. (1976): J. Am. Geriatr. Soc., 24:490-497.
93. Hyams, D.E. (1978): In: Textbook of Geriatric Medicine and Gerontology, pp. 670-711. Churchill Livingstone, New York.
94. Isogai, Y., Mochizuki, K., and Ashikago, M. (1981): Curr. Med. Res. Opin., 7:353-358.
95. Jarvik, M.E., Gritz, E.R., and Schneider, N.G. (1972): Behav. Biol., 7:643-668.
96. Jenden, D.J. (1979): In: Brain Acetylcholine and Neuropsychiatric Disease, edited by K.L. Davis and P.A. Berger, pp. 483-513. Plenum Press, New York.
97. Jotkowitz, S. (1983): Ann. Neurol., 14:690-691.
98. Kastin, A.J., Olson, R.D., Schally, A.V., and Coy, D.H. (1979): Life Sci., 25:401-414.

99. Knisely, M.H. (1965): In: Handbook of Physiology, The Circulation, edited by the American Physiological Society. pp. 2249-2292. Williams and Wilkins, Baltimore, Maryland.
100. Knisely, M.H., Bloch, E.H., Eliot, T.S., and Warner, L. (1947): Science, 106:431-440.
101. Koberle, S., and Spiegel, R. (1984): Gerontology, 30:3-52.
102. Kral, V.A. (1978): In: Alzheimer's Disease: Senile Dementia and Related Disorders, Vol. 7, edited by R. Katzman, R.D. Terry, and K.L. Bick, pp. 47-51. Raven Press, New York.
103. Krassner, M.B. (1984): Adv. Therapy, 3:172-189.
104. Kretschmar, J.H., and Kretschmar, C. (1976): Arzneim. Forsch., 26:1158-1159.
105. Kubanis, P., Gobbel, G., and Zornetzer, S.F. (1981): Behav. Neural Biol., 32:242-247.
106. Lehmann, E. (1984): Pharmacopsychiatr. Neuropsychopharmakol., 17:71-75.
107. Lehmann, H.E., and Ban, T.A. (1975): In: Genesis and Treatment of Psychological Disorders in the Elderly, Vol. 2, edited by S. Gershon, and A. Raskin, pp. 179-203. Raven Press, New York.
108. Lippa, A.S., Pelham, R.W., Beer, B., Critchett, D.J., Dean, R.L., and Bartus, R.T. (1980): Neurobiol. Aging, 1:13-20.
109. Lloyd-Evans, S., Brocklehurst, J.C., and Palmer, M.K. (1979): Curr. Med. Res. Opin., 6:351-357.
110. Loew, D.M. (1980): In: Aging of the Brain and Dementia, Vol. 12, edited by L. Amaducci, A.N. Davidson, and P. Antuono, pp. 287-294. Raven Press, New York.
111. Loew, D. (1984): Pharmacopsychiatr. Neuropsychopharmakol., 17:177.
112. Loveren-Huyben, C.M.S., Engelaar, H.F.W.J., Hermans, M.B.M., van der Bom, J.A., Leering, C., and Munnichs, J.M.A. (1984): J. Am. Geriatr. Soc., 32:584-588.
113. Malcolm, R., Bicher, H.I., Duncan, R.C., and Knisely, M.H. (1972): Microvasc. Res., 4:94-97.
114. Marriott, J.G., and Abelson, J.S. (1980): Age, 3:7-9.
115. Marriott, J.G., Bartus, R.T., Moyer, C., and Voigtman, R.E. (1979): Physiol. Behav., 22:715-722.
116. McDonald, R.J. (1979): Pharmakopsychiatr. Neuropsychopharmakol., 12:407-422.
117. McHenry, L.C. (1972): Stroke, 3:686-691.
118. Medin, D.L. (1969): Physiol. Psychol., 68:412-419.
119. Mindus, P., Cronholm, B., Levander, S.E., and Schalling, D., (1976): Acta Psychiatr. Scand., 54:150-160.
120. Miyamoto, M., Takayanagi, I., Ohkubo, H., and Takagi, K. (1976): Jpn. J. Pharmacol., 26:114-117.
121. Muller, R. (1979): J. Med., 10:307-329.

122. Muller, R., and Lehrach, F. (1980): Pharmatherapeutica, 2:372-379.
123. National Institute on Aging Task Force. (1980): JAMA, 244:259-263.
124. Nelson, J.J. (1975): Geriatrics, 30:133-142.
125. Nicolaus, B.J.R. (1982): Drug Dev., 2:463-474.
126. Office of Technology Assessment. (1985): Technology and Aging in America. OTA, Washington, D.C.
127. Ordy, J.M., and Brizzee, K.R., editors (1975): Advances in Behavioral Biology. Neurobiology of Aging: An Interdisciplinary Life-Span Approach, Vol. 16. Plenum Press, New York.
128. Oswald, W.D., Matejcek, M., Lukaschek, K., Dennler, H.J., and Oswald, B. (1982): Arzneim. Forsch., 32:584-590.
129. Panella, J.J., and Blass, J.P. (1984): Ann. Neurol., 15:308.
130. Perry, E.K. (1980): Age Ageing, 9:1-8.
131. Poech, G., and Kukovetz, W.R. (1971): Life Sci., 10:133-144.
132. Pomara, N., Reisberg, B., Ferris, S.H., and Gershon, S. (1981): In: Behavioral Assessment and Psychopharmacology, edited by F.J. Pirozzolo, and G.J. Maletta, pp. 107-143. Praeger Publishers, New York.
133. Pomara, N., Roberts, R., Rhiew, H.B., Stanley, M., and Gershon, S. (1985): Neurobiol. Aging, 6:233-236.
134. Prien, R.F. (1973): Psychopharmacol. Bull., 9:5-8.
135. Regli, R., Yamaguchi, T., and Waltz, A.G. (1971): Arch. Neurol., 24:467-474.
136. Reisberg, B., Ferris, S., Anand, R., Mir, P., Geiber, V., and DeLeon, M.J. (1983): N. Engl. J. Med., 308:721-722.
137. Rigter, H., and Crabbe, J.C. (1979): Vitam. Horm., 337:153-241.
138. Rosen, H.J. (1975): J. Am. Geriatr. Soc., 23:169-174.
139. Rosen, W.G., Mohs, R.C., and Davis, K.L. (1984): Am. J. Psychiatry, 141:1356-1364.
140. Rossor, M.N., Emson, P.C., Mountjoy, C.Q., Roth, M., and Iverson, L.L. (1980): Neurosci. Lett., 20:373-377.
141. Salzman, C., Kochansky, G.E., and Shader, R.I. (1972): Psychopharmacol. Bull., 8:3-50.
142. Samuel, D., Algeri, S., Gershon, S., Grimm, V.E., and Toffano, G., editors (1983): Aging of the Brain, Vol. 22. Raven Press, New York.
143. Scott, F.L. (1979): In: Physiology and Cell Biology of Aging, edited by A. Cherkin, C.E. Finch, N. Kharasch, T. Makinodan, F.L. Scott, and B.S. Strehler, pp. 151-184. Raven Press, New York.
144. Serby, M., Corwin, J., Rotrosen, J., Ferris, S.H., Reisberg, B., Friedman, E., Sherman, K.A., Jordan, B., and Bartus, R.T. (1983): Psychopharm. Bull., 19:126-129.

145. Shader, R.I., and Goldsmith, G.N. (1975): In: Progress in Psychiatric Drug Treatment, Vol. 2, edited by D.F. Klein and R. Gittleman-Klein. Brunner/Mazel, New York.
146. Simeon, J.G., Volavka, J., Trites, R., Waters, B., Webster, I., Ferguson, H.B., and Simeon, S. (1983): Psychopharmacol. Bull., 19:716-720.
147. Simeon, J., Waters, B., and Resnick, B. (1980): Psychopharmacol. Bull., 16:65-66.
148. Smith, C.M., and Swash, M. (1979): Lancet i:42.
149. Smith, R.C., Vroulis, G., Johnson, R., and Morgan, R. (1984): Psychopharm. Bull., 20:542-545.
150. Stegink, A.J. (1972): Arzneim. Forsch., 22:975-977.
151. Strong, R., Hicks, P., Hsu, L., Bartus, R.T., and Enna, S.J. (1980): Neurobiol. Aging, 1:59-63.
152. Strupp, B.J., and Levitsky, D.A. (1985): Neurosci. Biobehav. Rev., 9:399-411.
153. Strupp, B., Weingartner, H., Goodwin, F.K., and Gold, P.W. (1984): Pharmacol. Therapy, 23:179-191.
154. Terry, R., and Katzman, R. (1983): In: The Neurology of Aging, edited by R. Katzman and R. Terry, pp. 51-84. Davis, Philadelphia.
155. Thal, L.J., and Fuld, P.A. (1983): N. Engl. J. Med., 308:720.
156. Tomlinson, B.E., Blessed, G., and Roth, M. (1970): J. Neurol. Sci., 11:205-242.
157. U.S. Department of Health and Human Services. (1984): Alzheimer's Disease: Report of the Secretary's Task Force on Alzheimer's Disease. DHHS Publication No. (ADM) 84-1323.
158. Van Wimersma Greidanus, T.B., van Ree, J.M., and de Wied, D. (1983): Pharmacol. Ther., 20:437-458.
159. Volavka, J., Dornbush, R., Mallya, A., and Cho, D. (1979): Psychiatr. Res., 1:80-92.
160. Volavka, J., Simeon, J., Simeon, S., Cho, D., and Reker, D. (1981): Psychopharmacology, 72:185-188.
161. Walsh, A.C. (1969a): J. Am. Geriatr. Soc., 17:93-104.
162. Walsh, A.C. (1969b): J. Am. Geriatr. Soc., 17:477-487.
163. Weinberg, J. (1980): In: Comprehensive Textbook of Psychiatry, Vol. III, edited by H.I. Kaplan, A.M. Freedman, and B.J. Sadock, pp. 3024-3042. Williams & Wilkins, Baltimore, Maryland.
164. Whitehouse, P.J., Price, D.L., Clark, A.W., Coyle, J.T., and DeLong, M.R. (1981): Ann. Neurol., 10:122-126.
165. Wiegant, V.M., Zwiers, H., and Gispen, W.H. (1981): Pharmacol. Ther., 12:463-490.
166. Wilsher, C., Atkins, G., and Manfield, P. (1979): Psychopharmacology, 75:107-109.
167. Wurtman, R.J. (1979): In: Nutrition and the Brain, Choline and Lecithin in Brain Disorders, Vol. 5, edited by A. Barbeau, J.H. Growdon, and R.J. Wurtman, pp. 1-12. Raven Press, New York.

168. Yesavage, J.A. (1983): J. Am. Geriatr. Soc., 31:59-60.
169. Yesavage, J.A., Tinklenberg, J.R., Hollister, L.E., and Berger, P.A. (1979): Arch. Gen. Psychiatry, 36:220-223.
170. Yesavage, J.A., Westphal, J., and Rush, L. (1981): J. Am. Geriatr. Soc., 29:164-171.
171. Zelinsky, D. (1986): In: The Handbook of Clinical Memory Assessment in Older Adults, in press. American Psychological Association, Washington, D.C.

DRUG- AND ALCOHOL-INDUCED DEMENTIAS

Gerhard Freund

Endocrinology Section, Veterans Administration Medical Center
and University of Florida College of Medicine
Gainesville, Florida 32602

Dementia, as defined by the Diagnostic Statistical Manual III of Mental Disorders (DSM III), prepared by the American Psychiatric Association, is a loss of intellectual abilities involving memory, judgment, and abstract thought in the absence of delirium (reduced clarity of awareness of environment) and depression of mood (1). Table 1 lists functions which may be affected by organic dementia. The diagnosis of dementia is arrived at after other causes of reduced intellectual functioning are ruled out. Among other causes of impairment of intellectual abilities, drug- and alcohol-induced dementias are the most common.

TABLE 1. Dementia (definition, DSM III, 1980)

Loss of intellectual abilities
Memory (short-term, long-term)
Judgment
Abstract thought
Proverbs, similarities
Higher cortical functions
Sentence structure
Visuospacial
Personality changes

When depression (endogenous or drug-induced) interferes with intellectual function, it is called pseudodementia. A large number of drugs can temporarily reduce intellectual function by inducing either delirium (confusion) or emotional depression. This may be a primary effect of the drug or a side effect. Side effects resulting from the interaction between multiple drugs in the same elderly patient may include confusion or sedation which may be mistaken for organic dementias. When organic dementias (Alzheimer's disease, AD, or multi-infarct dementia, MID) and drug-induced pseudodementias coexist in the same person, the extent of the latter is evident from behavioral changes following the discontinuation of the causative drugs. Some classes of drugs produce symptoms of organic dementia by directly interfering with brain mechanisms of memory. Agents that produce these effects include corticosteroids (46) or anticholinergic agents (3,5,12). In Parkinson's disease, it may be difficult to separate these drug effects from those of the underlying brain disease (49).

In contrast to drugs in which the effects may mimic organic dementias, ethanol may induce a real organic dementia if consumed in large enough quantities. Chronic exposure to ethanol may cause intellectual impairment in the absence of thiamine deficiency (15). The severity of effects may range from global organic brain syndrome and Korsakoff's amnestic syndrome to milder forms of impairment which can be demonstrated only with sensitive neuropsychological tests (4,8,24,31,32). Most of these changes are permanent but some may be partially reversible with abstinence (10). These intellectual changes are moderately well-correlated with brain atrophy measured by CT scan (10). As with other drugs, the neurotoxicity of chronic alcohol exposure has been demonstrated in animals under genetically and nutritionally controlled conditions (15).

In the following sections, drug- and alcohol-induced dementia will be reviewed and discussed. The goal of this chapter is to describe the clinical features of these conditions and how they may be distinguished from Alzheimer's disease.

DEMENTIA

Cognitive function is defined as attention, language, memory, visuospacial and abstract reasoning. In its early stages, dementia may not be distinguishable from "benign senescent forgetfulness" (7,48). With normal aging, unimportant events may be forgotten. In contrast, forgetting of important events may indicate early dementia. As dementia progresses, some of the more difficult and sensitive neuropsychological tests may become abnormal. In contrast, the usual mental status examination (such as orientation in time and space) may be perfectly normal. As dementia progresses further, even these simple questions cannot be answered and the patient becomes "untestable" (25,30,33,41,45). Table 2 lists some of the types of memory testing.

The organic brain diseases which cause dementia (AD or MID) are not discussed here. It is important to distinguish drug-induced dementias and pseudodementias from these organic dementias in order to avoid unnecessary institutionalization

TABLE 2. Memory testing

---
       1. Immediate
          Digit span (six)
       2. Recent
          Five words or objects
       3. Remote
          Famous personalities
          Historical events
          Early experiences

---

and psychological trauma. Unlike the organic dementias, the drug-induced dementias are almost always reversible. However, sometimes both organic- and drug-induced dementias may coexist in the same patient. Furthermore, organic dementia may cause emotional depression which then further accentuates the features of true dementia.

CONFUSION, DELIRIUM

The DSM III lists the following diagnostic criteria:
A. Clouding of consciousness (reduced clarity of awareness of the environment), with reduced capacity to shift, focus, and sustain attention to environmental stimuli.
B. At least two of the following:
   1. perceptual disturbance: misinterpretations, illusions, or hallucinations
   2. speech that is at times incoherent
   3. disturbance of sleep-wakefulness cycle, with insomnia or daytime drowsiness
   4. increased or decreased psychomotor activity
C. Disorientation and memory impairment (if testable).
D. Clinical features that develop over a short period of time (usually hours to days) and tend to fluctuate over the course of a day.
Table 3 lists some of the main features of delirium:

TABLE 3. Delirium ("acute brain syndrome")

Reduction in the clarity of awareness of the environment
Decreased attention
Decreased perception
Decreased coherence of thought
Duration--weeks to one month
Susceptibility increased in senescence

A large number of drugs have been associated with delirium (49). Prominent among the elderly are cytostatic and immunosuppressive drugs used in cancer chemotherapy (38). They often cause depression of mood (36), delirium or both (38). This is probably part of a generalized neurotoxicity, and is particularly common after the use of 5-fluorouracie, L-asparaginase, methatrexate, nitrogen mustard and the vinca alkaloid related drugs.

DEPRESSION

The DSM III requires, for the diagnosis of depression, at least three of the following symptoms:
1. insomnia or hypersomnia
2. low energy level or chronic tiredness
3. feelings of inadequacy, loss of self-esteem, or self-deprecation
4. decreased effectiveness or productivity at school, work, or home
5. decreased attention, concentration, or ability to think clearly
6. social withdrawal
7. loss of interest in or enjoyment of pleasurable activities
8. irritability or excessive anger (in children, expressed toward parents or caretakers)
9. inability to respond with apparent pleasure to praise or rewards
10. less active or talkative than usual, or feels slowed down or restless
11. pessimistic attitude toward the future, brooding about past events, or feeling sorry for self
12. tearfulness or crying
13. recurrent thoughts of death or suicide

Table 4 lists the major features of general sedation induced by drugs, (left column). In addition, there may be symptoms of emotional depression listed in the right column.

TABLE 4. Effects of drug-induced sedation and symptoms of emotional depression

Sedation	Depressed mood
Apathy	Sedation plus:
Weakness	
Fatigue	Sadness
Drowsiness	Hopelessness
Sleepiness	Anxiety
Lethargy	Guilt
Decreased memory	Self-deprecation
Decreased cognition	Suicidal

Elderly patients with decreased renal function and increased sensitivity of the central nervous system to depressant drugs are particularly prone to drug-induced depression (36,48,49). Because of multiple diseases which require multiple medications, they are also more likely to be subject to multiple drug interactions which may induce sedation with dosages of drugs which are normally well-tolerated (36,49,52).

The most widely studied drug is the anticonvulsive phenytoin (dilantin®). This drug impairs memory only in very high doses and blood concentrations (14,43,44). Sedation may be enhanced by other antiepileptic drugs used in combination. Upon lowering the dose of phenytoin, impairment of cognitive function is usually reversible (42,43). However, it may not completely resolve because dementia may coexist as a result of pre-existing impairment or of the underlying seizure disorder.

Table 5 is a partial list of the sedatives which may induce pseudodementia. Various antihypertensive and benzodiazepines are often prescribed for the elderly (36). The antianxiety benzodiazepines are the currently, most widely prescribed group of drugs. Depression and sedation may occur in the elderly at a lower dosage level than that which induces these effects in younger persons (36). From 50-60 percent of elderly patients treated with antihypertensives may experience emotional depression (36).

TABLE 5. Drugs causing depression (pseudodementia) or exacerbating an existing depression

---

Alcohol
Antihistamines
Antihypertensives (reserpine, propranolol)
Anticancer
Antiparkinson
Antipsychotics (phenothiazines)
Cimetidine
Corticosteroids
Digitalis
Lithium
Narcotics
Sedatives--benzodiazepines, barbituates
                polypharmacy, drug interactions

Details of the differential diagnosis between pseudodementia and dementia are described elsewhere (12). Characteristically, patients with pseudodementia have a clear-cut onset, rapid progression, and are aware of and complain about the depression. Test performance is more variable with time, recognition is intact and learning a list of unrelated words is more impaired than learning a list of related words. Truly demented patients do poorly in learning both related and unrelated word lists. The depression may respond to tricyclic antidepressants, particularly those with low anticholinergic properties (5,12). Formal scales to quantify the degree of depression are available (52). They are useful to determine the effects of antidepressant drugs.

OTHER DRUG-INDUCED DEMENTIAS

Recently, a "dementia-like cognitive impairment" was described in patients receiving pharmacological doses of corticosteroids for systemic diseases (46). Deficits in memory, attention, concentration, mental speed and efficiency were observed. This syndrome was quite distinct from steroid psychoses. Several neuropsychological test scores were depressed during steroid therapy but invariably returned to normal several weeks after termination of corticosteroid therapy in all subjects.

Impairment of short-term memory has long been noticed following administration of scopolamine, a potent anticholinergic agent which crosses the blood-brain barrier. Subsequent controlled studies confirmed this effect and gave rise to the cholinergic hypothesis of memory formation and of cholinergic dysfunction in the elderly (3). Other drugs with anticholinergic side effects such as tricyclic antidepressants may be used for the treatment of depression in the elderly. The undesirable side effect of impairing memory in these patients can be avoided by selecting tricyclics with low intrinsic anticholinergic activity such as desipramine (12).

ALCOHOL-INDUCED DEMENTIA

Alcohol is the only drug that induces a dementia which may not be always reversible. The annual institutionalization rate for Korsakoff's amnestic syndrome is 8 per million adult population (11). Much more prevalent is a severe global dementia (24) (Dementia Associated with Alcoholism, 291.2x, DSM III). This dementia has the same clinical features as the other types of organic dementias (AD or MID). Many of these cases of end-stage alcohol dementia are in institutions where the diagnosis of alcoholism is often missed (2). Without an intensive search for a history of alcohol abuse, these patients are diagnosed as having Alzheimer's disease, multi-infarct dementia, or mixed dementias. The diagnosis of alcohol dementia is made in alcohol abusers by exclusion of other causes of organic dementias (1). Only further research can determine if this approach is correct because, potentially, alcohol abuse could be merely coincidental with other causes of dementia. A further major problem is that normal aging and age-related dementias, such as Alzheimer's disease and multi-infarct dementia, may coexist or interact with alcohol abuse (10,17,19,50). Alcoholism could be a risk factor for Alzheimer's disease.

The prevalence of alcohol abuse and any one of its medical consequences depends upon, first, how narrowly or broadly alcohol abuse and its consequences are defined. Second, the prevalence depends upon the sample population: those living in open community, medical outpatient, psychiatric outpatient, general hospital, mental institution, or nursing home, etc. For example, in state mental hospitals, approximately 9 percent of all admissions are for alcohol-related dementias, and in an additional 10 percent, alcohol-related diagnoses are missed unless special efforts are made to detect alcohol abuse in the past (2). In a sample of elderly first-admission psychiatric patients, 23 percent abused alcohol (39). Alcoholism-related admissions to Veterans Administration Medical Centers are in the range of 30 percent (29) and as many as 50 percent of patients abuse alcohol even though this abuse is not directly responsible for the admission (22). Very little is currently known about the extent and type of problem drinking in the elderly population living in open communities (23,28,40,49). However, two types of alcohol abuse appear to be distinguishable: survivors of long-term alcohol abuse and those who begin alcohol abuse in their old age ("secondary alcoholics").

Alcohol abuse may be defined either by its causes (amount of alcohol consumed), or by its consequences (impairment of social function, physical or mental health), or both. No quantitative data are available regarding the amounts of alcohol that must be consumed in order to cause dementia. However, the amounts of alcohol listed in Table 6 indicate the consumption associated with damage to tissues other than the brain.

Not all heavy drinkers become demented. The question is what genetic and/or environmental factors render susceptible to or protect against the effects of chronic alcohol abuse on the brain. There is some evidence that genetic factors influence the causes, the predisposition to alcohol abuse (18), but little is known about genetic factors which may determine the consequences, such as the severity of alcohol-induced encephalopathy. Such genetic factors could make individuals more vulnerable to the effects of alcohol by virtue of increased susceptibility of specific tissues, specific cells, or enzymes. Of the environmental factors, absolute alcohol consumption (daily amounts, total lifetime amounts, distribution of alcohol consumption, duration, age at onset, etc.), nutritional factors, exposure to industrial chemicals or toxins, use of other drugs or currently unknown conditions could play a role in determining the degree of neurotoxicity of alcohol. For example, it is well-established that thiamine deficiency causes Wernicke's encephalopathy (32). It has been found that an abnormality of a thiamine-requiring enzyme

TABLE 6. Alcohol consumption of alcohol users and abusers

Author	Ref No.[a]	E/day[b]	E/kg[c]	Liters/Year	Duration	Tissue
NCA	13	280	3.4	130	2 days	--
Schmidt & de Lint	37	120-270	--	55-125	--	--
Whalley	47	120-400	--	55-180	--	--
Lelbach	27	120-270	--	55-125	5 yr	Liver
Klatsky et al.	26	40	--	18	--	Heart
Yano et al.	51	50	--	23	--	Heart
Carey et al.	9	50-80	--	23-36	12 day	Blood Chemistry

[a]The first four references indicate that these amounts of alcohol may be associated with alcohol-induced impairment. The amounts investigated in the last three references of the table have not been associated with significant illness. In analogy to nicotine abuse where cigarette consumption is expressed as pack-years (packs of cigarettes per day times years of abuse), alcohol abuse could be expressed as hectogram-years (1 hg = 100 g) or pint-years (150 g ethanol) of absolute alcohol consumption.
[b]E = absolute ethanol in grams (1 ml = 0.8 gm)
[c]E/kg = E/kg body weight/day

predisposes to the development of this encephalopathy (6). It is controversial whether or not Wernicke's encephalopathy is the direct cause of Korsakoff's amnestic syndrome or merely an association in those alcohol abusers who are also malnourished (15,20). However, this example demonstrates how genetic and environmental factors could interact to cause a disease.

There are several mechanisms whereby alcohol abuse could impair cognitive function ranging from mild impairment to dementia (16,20,21). First, alcohol, like other neurotoxic substances, could directly destroy neurons and/or their associated synapses. This results in gross, diffuse atrophy demonstrable by CT scans (10). Second, alcoholics are subject to the same spectrum of brain diseases as nonalcoholics in the general population (20). For example, alcoholics are more prone to head trauma, subdural hematomas and cerebrovascular accidents. Nothing is currently known about alcohol abuse as a risk factor in Alzheimer's disease or multi-infarct dementia. Third, normal aging may cause mild impairment of cognitive function. It has been well-established by many investigators that controls for age must be established whether they measure brain atrophy by CT scan (10) or performance by neuropsychological test batteries (4,31,34,35,50).

CONCLUSIONS

Drug-induced dementias may be mistaken for organic dementias such as Alzheimer's disease or multi-infarct dementia. Because virtually all drug-induced dementias are reversible, it is essential to have a high index of suspicion. Organic and drug-induced dementias may coexist in the same patient, and early organic dementia may cause emotional depression. Drugs may induce a reversible dementia (pseudodementia) by precipitating confusion, delirium, sedation, or emotional depression. Certain clinical features and a response to treatment with antidepressants suggest that the dementia is drug-induced rather than organic.

Alcohol abuse may cause various degrees of mild impairment of cognitive function, amnestic (Korsakoff's) syndrome, and global dementias clinically indistinguishable from other organic dementias. The alcohol-related dementias are only partially reversible in some patients. The diagnosis of alcohol dementia is frequently missed in institutionalized patients. Alcohol abuse may coexist in the same patient with other disorders causing dementia. Impairment of cognitive function with normal aging may be worsened by alcohol abuse in an additive or potentiating fashion. The aged brain may be more susceptible to the neurotoxic effects of alcohol. The role of alcohol abuse as a risk factor in Alzheimer's disease and multi-infarct dementia is currently unknown.

REFERENCES

1. American Psychiatric Association, Diagnostic Statistical Manual of Mental Disorders (DSM III), ed. 3. (1980): American Psychiatric Association, Evanston, Illinois.
2. Bachrach, L.L. (1976): In: NIMH Mental Health Statistical Note, No. 124, Feb. U.S. Government Printing Office, Washington, D.C.
3. Bartus, R.T., Dean, R.L., III, Beer, B., and Lippa, A.S. (1982): Science, 217:408-417.
4. Becker, J.T., Butters, N., Hermann, A., and D'Angelo, N. (1983): Alcoholism: Clin. Exp. Res., 7:213-219.
5. Bernstein, J.G. (1984): J. Clin. Psychiatry, 45:30-34.
6. Blass, J.P., and Gibson, G.E. (1977): N. Engl. J. Med., 297:1367-1370.
7. Branconnier, J., and DeVitt, D.R. (1983): In: Alzheimer's Disease, edited by B. Reisberg, pp. 214-227. The Free Press, New York.
8. Butters, N., and Cermak, L.S. (1980): Alcoholic Korsakoff's Syndrome. An Information-Processing Approach to Amnesia. Academic Press, New York.
9. Carey, M.A., Jones, J.D., Gastineau, C.F. (1971): JAMA, 216:1766-1769.

10. Carlen, P.L., Wortzman, G., Holgate, R.C., Wilkinson, D.A., and Rankin, J.G. (1978): Science, 200:1076-1078.
11. Centerwall, B.S., and Criqui, M.H. (1978): N. Engl. J. Med., 299:285-289.
12. Cole, J.O., Branconnier, R., Salomon, M., and Dessain, E. (1983): J. Clin. Psychiatry, 44:14-19.
13. Criteria Committee, National Council on Alcoholism (1972): Ann. Intern. Med., 77:249-258.
14. Dodrill, C.B. (1975): Epilepsia, 16:593-600.
15. Freund, G. (1973): Annu. Rev. Pharmacol., 13:217-227.
16. Freund, G. (1982): In: Alcoholism and Aging: Advances in Research, edited by W.G. Wood and M.F. Elias, pp. 131-148. CRC Press, Boca Raton.
17. Freund, G. (1982): Alcoholism: Clin. Exp. Res., 6:13-21.
18. Freund, G. (1984): Alcohol, 1:129-131.
19. Freund, G. (1984): In: Recent Developments in Alcoholism, Volume II, edited by M. Galanter, pp. 65-83. Plenum Press, New York.
20. Freund, G. (1985): In: Alcohol and the Brain, edited by R.E. Tarter and D.H. VanThiel, pp. 3-17. Plenum Press, New York.
21. Freund, G., and Butters, N. (1982): Alcoholism: Clin. Exp. Res., 6:1-2.
22. Gomberg, E.S. (1975): J. Stud. Alcohol, 36:1458-1467.
23. Hartford, J.T., and Samorajski, T. (1984): Alcoholism in the Elderly: Social and Biomedical Issues. Raven Press, New York.
24. Horvath, T.B. (1975): In: Alcohol, Drugs, and Brain Damage, edited by J.G. Rankin, pp. 1-16. Alcoholism and Drug Addiction Research Foundation of Ontario, Toronto.
25. Katzman, R., Terry, R.D., and Bick, K.L. (1978): Alzheimer's Disease: Senile Dementia and Related Disorders. Raven Press, New York.
26. Klatsky, A.L., Friedman, G.D., Siegelaub, A.B. (1974): Ann. Intern. Med., 81:294-301.
27. Lelbach, W.K. (1974): In: Research Advances in Alcohol and Drug Problems, edited by R.J. Gibbins, Y. Israel, H. Kalant, R.E. Popham, W. Schmidt, and R.G. Smart, pp. 93-198. John Wiley, New York.
28. Maddox, G., Robins, L.N., and Rosenberg, N., editors (1984): Research Monograph No. 14. Nature and Extent of Alcohol Problems Among the Elderly. National Institute on Alcohol Abuse and Alcoholism, Rockville, Maryland.
29. McAllister, R.G., Jr., and Dzur, J. (1974): Southern Med. J., 67:388-392.
30. McKhann, G., Drachman, D., Folstein, M., Katzman, R., Price, D., and Stadlan, E. (1984): Neurology, 34:939-944.
31. Parsons, O.A., and Farr, S.P. (1981): In: Handbook of Clinical Neuropsychology, edited by S.B.F. Felskon and T.J. Bolls, pp. 320-365. John Wiley, New York.

32. Phillips, G.B., Victor, M., Adams, R.D., and Davidson, C.S. (1952): J. Clin. Invest., 31:859-871.
33. Reisberg, B., editor (1983): Alzheimer's Disease. The Free Press, New York.
34. Riege, W.H., Tomaszewski, R., Lanto, A., and Metter, E.J. (1984): Alcoholism: Clin. Exp. Res., 8:42-47.
35. Ryan, C. (1982): Alcoholism: Clin. Exp. Res., 6:22-30.
36. Salzman, C., and Shader, R.I. (1978): J. Am. Geriatr. Soc., 26:303-308.
37. Schmidt, W., and de Lint, J. (1970): Q. J. Stud. Alcohol, 31:957-964.
38. Silberfarb, P.M. (1983): Annu. Rev. Med., 34:35-46.
39. Simon, A., Epstein, L.J., and Reynolds, L. (1968): Geriatrics, 23:125-131.
40. Tabakoff, B., Sutker, P.B., and Randall, C.L., editors (1983): Medical and Social Aspects of Alcohol Abuse. Plenum Press, New York.
41. Terry, R.D., and Davies, P. (1980): Annu. Rev. Neurosci., 3:77-95.
42. Thompson, P. J., and Trimble, M.R. (1982): Epilepsia, 23:531-544.
43. Trimble, M.R. (1981): Curr. Dev. Psychopharmacol., 6:65-91.
44. Trimble, M.R., and Reynolds, E.H. (1976): Psychol. Med., 6:169-178.
45. U.S. Dept. of Health and Human Services (1984): Report of the Secretary's Task Force on Alzheimer's Disease. Washington, D.C.
46. Varney, N.R., Alexander, B., and MacIndoe, J.H. (1984): Am. J. Psychiatry, 141:369-372.
47. Whalley, L.J. (1979): J. Stud. Alcohol, 40:117-119.
48. Whelihan, W.M., Lesher, E.L., Kleban, M.H., and Granick, S. (1984): J. Gerontol., 39:572-576.
49. Whittington, F.J. (1983): In: Drugs and the Elderly Adult, edited by M.D. Glantz, D.M. Petersen, and F.J. Whittington, pp. 203-206. ADAMHA Research Issues 32, Rockville, Maryland.
50. Wood, W.G., and Elias, M.F., editors. (1982): Alcoholism and Aging: Advances in Research. CRC Press, Boca Raton.
51. Yano, K., Rhoads, G.G., and Kagan, A. (1977): N. Engl. J. Med., 297:405-409.
52. Yesavage, J.A., Brink, T.L., Rose, L., and Adey, M. (1983): In: Assessment in Geriatric Psychopharmacology, edited by T. Crook, S. Ferris, and R. Bartus, pp. 153-165. Mark Powley Associates, New Canaan, Connecticut.

IMPACT OF AGING ON HOST RESPONSE TO INFECTIOUS DISEASE

Thomas T. Yoshikawa

Geriatric Research, Education, and Clinical Center,
Veterans Administration Medical Center, Wadsworth Division,
and Department of Medicine, UCLA School of Medicine,
Los Angeles, California 90073

Infectious diseases are now recognized as important causes of serious morbidity and mortality in the geriatric population (19). Thus, the diagnosis, treatment, and prevention of infections in the elderly are important clinical problems for physicians and other health care professionals (21). However, the host-parasite (person-infecting pathogen) interaction varies considerably depending on whether the host is elderly or a younger adult. Age differences in the host-parasite are attributed in a large part to six important factors. These factors are: 1) frequency of morbidity and mortality due to infections; 2) susceptibility to and host defense mechanisms against infections; 3) clinical manifestations of infections; 4) etiology of certain infectious diseases; 5) response to chemotherapy; and 6) response to and effectiveness of immunoprophylaxis. This chapter will survey these factors with respect to aging and infectious diseases.

MORBIDITY AND MORTALITY

Not all infectious diseases have been shown to have dire consequences in old people. However, the relatively more common infectious diseases appear to be important in the geriatric age group (18). Table 1 compares the mortality rates of the average adult population versus the geriatric population for select infectious diseases. There are probably multiple factors that contribute to higher death rates from these infections in the elderly. These factors most likely include: 1) lack of adequate physiological reserve capacity in various organs and organ systems (e.g., cardiovascular); 2) compromised host defense mechanisms; 3) presence of chronic (and acute) underlying illnesses; 4) greater exposure to virulent pathogens (more hospitalization and chronic antibiotic use); 5) delays in

TABLE 1. Mortality from select infections in the general versus the geriatric population

	Mortality (%)		
Infection	General Population	Geriatric Population	Reference
Acute pneumonia	8[a]	39[a]	15
Pneumococcal pneumonia[b]	13[c]	53[c]	9
Tuberculosis	0.0002-0.0018[d]	0.007-0.015[d]	8
Acute cholecystitis	3[e]	3-24[e]	4
Acute appendicitis	1.0-1.0[f]	2.0-14.0[f]	13
Infective endocarditis	8.5[f]	21[f]	2
Staphylococcal endocarditis	41[g]	84[g]	16
Gram-negative bacillary sepsis	26[h]	70[h]	7
Bacterial meningitis	13[i]	41[i]	6

[a]Under the age of 40 years and 70 years and older
[b]Bacteremic cases
[c]Under age 50 years and 70 years and older
[d]Age 15-54 years and 65-85 and older
[e]Under age 65 years and 65-74 and 75 and older
[f]Under age 60 years and 60 years and older
[g]Under age 50 years and 50 years and older (21 of 37 patients 70 years and older)
[h]Age 16-55 years and 55 years and older
[i]Age 15-49 years and 50 years and older (mean age 64 years)

diagnosis and treatment; 6) poorer tolerance to invasive diagnosis and therapeutic procedures (e.g., surgery); 7) delay in response to antibiotic therapy; and 8) higher incidence of adverse effects of antibiotic therapy.

Similarly, morbidity rates are higher in the elderly, presumably related to the same factors that contribute to higher mortality. For example, appendicitis, which occurs both in the young and the aged, has a morbidity rate of 3-8 percent in the younger patient compared to 35-65 percent in the elderly patient (11). Bacteremia, as a complication of acute pyelonephritis, occurs with low frequency in young women but rises to an incidence of nearly 50 percent in elderly women (5). More importantly, bacteremia associated with shock occurs three to four times more frequently in the elderly compared to young adults (17).

SUSCEPTIBILITY AND HOST DEFENSES TO INFECTION

Like mortality, the higher susceptibility of the aged person to many infectious diseases is related to several factors (21). For a susceptible host to become infected, he/she must be exposed to potential pathogens. Chronic hospitalization predisposes to colonization with nosocomial organisms. Certainly, old patients are hospitalized more frequently and for longer periods. Thus, it is not surprising that the nosocomial infection rate in the elderly is three times higher than the general population (3). The presence of certain underlying chronic diseases may increase the susceptibility to various infectious diseases. These include malignancies (and associated treatment modalities), collagen vascular disease, diabetes mellitus, chronic obstructive lung disease, obstructive uropathy, and aspiration syndromes (e.g., stroke). Most, if not all, of these conditions occur predominantly in the middle- and old-aged person. The physiological changes that occur with normal aging generally cause decremental changes in organ function and reserve capacities. These organ system changes with aging as well as aberrations in the host defense mechanisms found in the elderly most likely contribute to a greater predisposition to select infections.

The host defense system (i.e., mechanical barriers, phagocytosis, and immune system) is affected to varying degrees by advancing age. Skin and mucus membranes do become less resistant to infection with age. Both the immune function of T lymphocytes (cell-mediated immunity) and humoral immunity clearly declines in the aged. Phagocytosis may be normal or minimally affected in old people. The impact of age on interferons, natural killer cells, and secretory immunity is still unclear (19).

CLINICAL MANIFESTATIONS OF INFECTION

The clinical manifestations of infections in the elderly may be quite variable (20). The clinical features may be classic for a focal infection; symptoms and signs may be atypical; or the patient may be minimally symptomatic or exhibit no symptoms referable to a particular infection. Several factors contribute to the unpredictable nature of clinical expression of disease, including infections, in the old (14). These include: 1) underreporting of symptoms by the elderly which may be related to ethnic, educational, or cultural background, cognitive impairment, denial, or depression; and 2) altered responses to infection which may be influenced by the biological changes of aging, coexisting chronic diseases, and differences in biological expression of diseases.

A common manifestation of infection (as well as of any disease or change of health status) in the old is alteration in mental status or cognitive function. Additionally, malaise, weakness, anorexia, weight loss, or nausea may be the only symptoms of infection in this population. Fever, a hallmark of infection, may be blunted or absent in the elderly (21). Although the precise pathogenetic mechanism for this fever abnormality has not been defined, preliminary animal data suggest that aging may alter the host's own endogenous pyrogen or the host's ability to adequately respond to endogenous pyrogen (10).

ETIOLOGY OF INFECTIONS

The bacterial etiology of common infectious disease syndromes in the old may deviate or be quite diverse from the typical bacterial causes seen in younger adults. Awareness and knowledge of these differences are especially important when decisions have to be made on antibiotic treatment in the elderly under circumstances in which: 1) a specific etiology cannot be determined; or 2) the patient is ill enough to warrant empiric treatment before microbiological data can become available.

Table 2 lists some infectious disease syndromes and the differences in bacteriologic etiology that may be seen in

TABLE 2.   Etiological differences of bacterial infections in the elderly

Infection	Common etiology in adults	Common etiology in elderly
Community-acquired pneumonia	Streptococcus pneumoniae	S. pneumoniae, Hemophilus influenzae, Staphylococcus aureus, Legionella sp. or gram-negative bacilli
Urinary tract infection (non-catheterized)	Escherichia coli	E. Coli, Proteus sp., Klebsiela sp., other gram-negative bacilli; or enterococci
Infective endocarditis (Natural valve, nondrug addict)	Viridans group streptococci	Viridans group streptococci, S. bovis, enterococci or S. aureus
Meningitis	S. pneumoniae, Neisseria meningitidis	S. pneumoniae, Listeria monocytogenes, gram-negative bacilli
Septic arthritis	N. gonorrhoeae	S. aureus, streptococci, or gram-negative bacilli

elderly patients (12,21). The pathogenetic factors that might explain these etiological differences are unclear. Presence of underlying diseases, chronic hospitalization, prolonged use of antibiotics, differences in host susceptibility, invasive diagnostic procedures or surgery may be contributory factors.

RESPONSE TO CHEMOTHERAPY

There are few, if any, data adequately comparing the response to antibiotics patients with that of younger adults who have the same infection. The author's clinical experience suggests that older patients have more delayed responses (using fever, clinical well-being, and microbial eradication as parameters) to antibiotic therapy than younger persons. (In some instances, they fail to respond despite appropriate therapy). However, this empiric observation may be influenced by several other factors that are unique to the elderly, i.e., diminished organ perfusion (due to arteriosclerosis or diabetes mellitus) and changes in organ function because of aging, both of which influence drug pharmacology, higher rates of drug side effects (limiting the dose of drug that can be given), and altered host defense mechanisms (which might be further compromised in the presence of active infection). These factors most certainly will influence the host response to antibiotic therapy.

RESPONSE TO IMMUNOPROPHYLAXIS

Prevention of infection certainly is the most optimal and cost-effective approach to managing infectious diseases in the elderly. One approach, though currently limited in scope, is to provide immunoprophylaxis (vaccination) for the elderly against select infections. The available vaccines that are recommended for the aged include tetanus toxoid, influenza virus, and pneumococcal polysaccharide. However, several studies indicate that the elderly have depressed immunological response compared to younger adults when given the vaccine antigens (1). The antibody responses in the old fail to achieve levels that are seen in middle-aged adults. It appears that functional abnormalities in T lymphocytes (helper cells) that modulate B lymphocyte activity are in part responsible for this aberration. Although protective antibody titers appear to be adequate for the elderly when immunized with antigen against tetanus, influenza, and pneumococcal disease (1), it has not been shown that these vaccines are as efficacious in the aged as in younger adults.

CONCLUSION

Infections must always be considered as a potential cause for a change in health status or well-being of an older person. Delays in diagnosis and proper treatment for an infection will lead to high mortality and morbidity in the elderly. Atypical or nonspecific clinical manifestations, varied and diverse etiologies, risks of diagnostic procedures, and suboptimal response to chemotherapy must be always considered in the management of the geriatric patient with a potential infectious disease illness. Optimally, prevention will be the most effective approach in decreasing patient suffering and reducing the enormous costs of treating infections in the elderly.

REFERENCES

1. Bentley, D.W. (1984): In: Immunology and Infectious Diseases in the Elderly, edited by R.A. Fox, pp. 333-370, Churchill Livingstone, Edinburg.
2. Cantrell, M. and Yoshikawa, T.T. (1983): J. Am. Geriatr. Soc., 31:216-222.
3. Freeman, J., and McGowan, J.E., Jr., (1973): J. Infect. Dis., 133:811-819.
4. Fry, D.E., Cox, R.A., and Harbrecht, J.P. (1981): South. Med. J., 74:666-668.
5. Gleckman, R.A., Bradley, P.J., Roth, R.M., and Hibert, D.M. (1985): J. Urol., 133:174-175.
6. Gorse, G.J., Thrupp, L.D., Nudleman, K.L., Wyle, F.A., Hawkins, B., and Cesario, T.C. (1984): Arch. Intern. Med., 144:1603-1607.
7. Hodgin, U.G., and Sanford, J.P. (1965): Am. J. Med., 39:952-960.
8. Meyers, J.A. (1976): Am. J. Public Health, 66:1101-1106.
9. Mufson, M.A., Kruss, D.M., Wasil, R.E., and Metzger, W.I. (1974): Arch. Intern. Med., 134:505-510.
10. Norman, D.C., Cantrell, M., Ngo, D., and Yoshikawa, T.T. (1984): Fed. Proc., 14:1828.
11. Norman, D.C., and Yoshikawa, T.T. (1983): J. Am. Geriatr. Soc., 31:677-684.
12. Norman, D.C., and Yoshikawa, T.T. (1983): Geriatrics, 38:83-91.
13. Norman, D.C., and Yoshikawa, T.T. (1984): J. Gerontol., 30:327-338.
14. Norman, D.C., and Yoshikawa, T.T. (1986): In: Infectious Diseases in the Elderly, edited by B.A. Cunha, in press. John Wright and Co., London.
15. Sullivan, R.J., Jr., Dowdle, W.R., Marine, W.M., and Hierholzer, J.C. (1972): Arch. Intern. Med., 129:935-942.
16. Watanakunakorn, C., Tan, J.C., and Phair, J.P. (1973): Am. J. Med., 54:473-481.
17. Weil, M.H., Shubin, H., and Biddle, M. (1964): Ann. Intern. Med., 60:384-400.
18. Yoshikawa, T.T. (1982): West. J. Med., 135:441-445.
19. Yoshikawa, T.T. (1984): J. Gerontol., 30:275-278.

20. Yoshikawa, T.T. (1985): In: Principles and Practice of Geriatric Medicine, edited by M.S.J. Pathy, pp. 221-238. John Wiley and Sons, Ltd., London.
21. Yoshikawa, T.T., Norman, D.C., and Grahn, D. (1985): J. Am. Geriatr. Soc., 33:496-503.

HOST DEFENSES AND THE ANTIBIOTIC TREATMENT OF PNEUMONIA IN THE ELDERLY

Ian M. Smith and Todd P. Semla*

Department of Internal Medicine,
University of Iowa Hospitals and Clinics,
Iowa City, Iowa 52242; and *Geriatric Pharmacotherapy,
College of Pharmacy, University of Iowa, Iowa City, Iowa 52242

There are many physiological changes in the lung that accompany aging, but it is apparent that diseases which affect the lung overshadow to some degree these physiological changes in predisposing to pneumonia. However, if we consider that at age 60, there are 110 females alive for every 100 males, and at age 80, there are 227 females for every 100 males, something lethal is happening to the aging male. We suggest that one of the important things happening is the development of pneumonia (7,78,82,86).

Autopsy studies in the nursing home and hospital show a high prevalence of pneumonia. Pneumonia as the primary cause of death in long-term care is somewhere between 13 to 15 percent; in an additional 20 percent, it is the secondary cause; and it is the cause of death in six to eight percent in acute care hospitals (40,44,49,62). Nonautopsy studies utilizing death certificates are only 50 percent accurate, and one gets the erroneous impression that cerebral vascular disease is high on the list. If one separates out different types of cancer, the number one cause of death in the elderly at autopsy is myocardial infarction which is statistically different from the causes of death in younger adults in the age group 30 to 49 (Table 1). No other cause of death is statistically different. The number two and three causes of death are septicemia and pneumonia as diagnosed by the pathologist (Table 1).

The incidence of lobar or pneumococcal pneumonia increases linearly starting at age 30 (42). Therefore, there is a very high incidence in elderly patients. Macfarlane et al. (53), in Nottingham, England, used counter-immune-electrophoresis in an attempt to diagnose otherwise undiagnosable pneumonia cases. Other studies demonstrated that 57 percent of the cases were due to pneumococci and 30 percent were due to an unknown cause (22). Case fatality rate in the unknown causes, however, was

TABLE 1. Primary and secondary causes of death at autopsy[a]
University of Iowa Hospitals 1973-1979

361 deaths at age 30-49	%	443 deaths at age 70 and over	%
All types of cancer	34	All types of cancer	30
Septicemia	17	Myocardial infarction	15
Cirrhosis	10	Septicemia	15
Pneumonia	10	Pneumonia	13
Leukemia	8	Postoperative complications	13
Postoperative complications	9	Leukemia	8
Myocardial infarction	7[b]	Pulmonary embolus	7
		Cardiac failure	6

[a]Reference 80
[b]$p < .01$

similar to the pneumococcal disease. The Nottingham group showed that they could make a definite diagnosis of the etiology of pneumonia in 98 percent of cases. Seventy-five percent of pneumonia is pneumococcal (Table 2).

Nursing home pneumonias (32,70) may be similar to community pneumonias if antibiotic usage is low. When nursing home residents are admitted to a general hospital, the pneumonias tend to be caused by antibiotic-resistant Klebsiella pneumoniae or Staphylococcus aureus two to four times as frequently as in similar aged community dwellers. Such patients are eight times as likely to have received prior antibiotics as are elderly community patients admitted to the hospital with pneumonia. Such pneumonias in the elderly are 40 percent fatal, compared to 20 percent in community-acquired pneumonias. This high fatality rate is underscored by the finding of pneumonia in 41 percent of autopsies in nursing home residents. In view of these pathogens, nursing home patients with pneumonia who are admitted to the hospital should be treated with cefuroxime, cefamandole, or trimethoprim-sulfamethoxazole. Many of these patients have underlying emphysema, influenza, alcoholism, aspiration, or congestive cardiac failure, and have prior pharyngeal colonization with antibiotic-resistant, gram-negative rods. Tuberculosis must always be ruled out, as 29 percent of new cases of pulmonary tuberculosis comes from the elderly

TABLE 2. Pneumonia classification and prognosis in patients age 65 and older[a]

Causative agent	Etiology (%)	Case fatality rate (%)
Pneumococci	72	14
Gram-negative rods	21	70
Legionella	5	10
All others	2	2

[a]Adapted from references 22 and 54

population. Lack of response to treatment in 24 to 48 hours should always indicate the need for acute care hospital transfers. Nursing home patients require pneumococcal vaccination and yearly influenza vaccine to avoid these lethal diseases.

PREDISPOSITION TO PNEUMONIA

Changes Due to Aging

Many changes occur in the structure of the lung with aging. These are summarized in Table 3 (79). The Framington study indicated that the best way to measure physiological aging in the lung is forced expiratory volume in one second (FEV_1) correlated with height. Table 4 shows mortality according to vital capacity index by age group and sex. A practicing clinician can use these data as a biological marker of aging in patients (47).

TABLE 3. Lung changes with age[a]

Structural	Calcified costal cartilages, kyphosis, decreased elastic fiber
Biochemical	Mucopolysaccharides, electrolytes
Immunologic	Decreased IgM, increased IgE, decreased thymus, decreased delayed sensitivity, polymorphonuclear leukocyte changes
Volumes	Decreased MBC, decreased FVC, decreased FEV, decreased VC, increased RV, increased lung compliance with decreased chest wall compliance
Gas exchange	Decreased ventilation with increased $PaCO_2$ and decreased PaO_2
Exercise	Capacity decreased with age; training may improve
Mechanical	Indwelling tubes and tracheostomy; cough reflex decreased
Thermal	20 percent have no fever with pneumonia
Measure	FVC related to height

[a]Reference 79

Underlying Disease States

A study from Milwaukee by Ebright and Rytel (22) shows that the elderly have significant underlying disease states in 85 percent, in contrast to the younger age groups where the figures are considerably lower. Comorbid diseases should be diagnosed promptly, because one-half of patients with pneumonia die of the pneumonia, but the other half die of ensuing failure in some other organ system which was borderline before the energy was used up to combat the pneumonia.

The attack rate by age for influenza B doubles from young adults to the elderly. Although we detect five to ten percent of a family practice with influenza during an outbreak, there are 40 percent of people in nursing homes involved. Although only one percent of these develop pneumonia, it becomes a significant number in nursing homes due to the high influenza attack rate. Adenovirus infection can also predispose to pneumonia (24).

TABLE 4. Mortality according to vital capacity index (VCI) 20-year followup, age 45 to 74

Annual Mortality			
Men		Women	
VCI (ml/inch)	Mortality Rate/1000	VCI (ml/inch)	Mortality Rate/1000
12-43	30	12-35	13
44-55	14	36-43	7
56-85	9	44-85	4

Admissions to the acute care hospital since the onset of Medicare have gone up eight percent for all age groups, but for people aged 65 and over, admissions have increased 38 percent. Therefore, we are admitting a lot of elderly people to the acute care hospital, and pneumonia is one of the significant nosocomial infections. Nosocomial infection rates rise astronomically as the age goes up. A history of previous hospitalization is also a risk factor for developing pneumonia (29).

DIAGNOSIS

An acceptable pneumonia classification is shown in Table 2. Lobar pneumonia (or pneumococcal pneumonia) is by far the most common. Staphylococcal pneumonia is rare, except in newborn children and in the aged, particularly following a flu epidemic. Mycoplasmal pneumonia is a disease of school-age children and their young parents, and we see it only rarely in the elderly. Gram-negative rod pneumonia is very important to characterize and is institutionally acquired. We used to say hospital acquired, but we now find a lot of them coming from the nursing home. A special brand of gram-negative rod pneumonia, Legionella pneumonia, particularly afflicts the elderly (43,54). Aspiration pneumonia affects people who are damaged in swallowing mechanisms or in brain function with problems with swallowing.

A study combining the results from Milwaukee (22) and the results from Nottingham (53) is shown in Table 2. Pneumococcal pneumonia comprises 75 percent. The case fatality rate (the number of deaths per hundred cases) on the right is 14 percent. A smaller percentage have gram-negative rod pneumonia, but is very much more lethal (70 percent). The Legionella pneumonia is not as lethal as other gram-negative rods. All the other pneumonias together are not very important. Basically, we are trying to prevent and treat pneumococcal pneumonia and to prevent and treat gram-negative rod pneumonia in the elderly (7,9,10). Blood cultures should be taken (approximately 25 percent of pneumonias are complicated by a positive blood culture), as this will change the prognosis and will make your care of this patient more intensive (20).

Factors Affecting Diagnosis

In general, history and physical examinations are very important (25). Middle-aged adults will report that they were well until the night before and they woke up in the middle of the night coughing up bloody or rusty sputum, and that every time they coughed or took a deep breath, there was stabbing (pleuritic) pain. They had a shivering attack at onset, then a temperature of 102° F, or higher. With these symptoms, pneumonia is not hard to diagnose. In the elderly, many of these symptoms may be absent, but the constant thing is the respiratory rate. We should be counting respiratory rates more often in the nursing homes. A fairly high percentage of people with increased respiratory rates over 26 have abnormalities on chest x-ray (92). All of them should be x-rayed, but most nursing homes are not equipped with x-ray machines. It is expensive and difficult to get elderly patients to acute facilities and get a chest x-ray. Therefore, physicians are tempted and do use empirical treatment; empirical treatment is often incorrect and leads to unnecessary deaths. The young may present with pleurisy, but approximately 20 percent of the elderly do not. Many of them just get confused. One must get a proper specimen of sputum (25 or more pus cells per high power field). Without this, you cannot make a proper diagnosis. A blood culture is also necessary, as 25 percent of the elderly pneumonia patients are septicemic.

Another factor is change in temperature. In general terms, 10 to 20 percent of elderly people that have infections have no fever (78). A study of the maximum temperature in response to bacteremia in different age groups has been done in relation to creatinine clearance (by measuring the area under the curve of the temperature chart and also measuring the mean maximum temperature) (89). There are significant differences as age advances. People with renal disease have less fever and many elderly people have chronic renal failure (89).

In addition to temperature regulation being impaired in some elderly, 50 percent of elderly people who have a serious infection have no rise in the total white count, but in 95 percent, the differential white count has shifted to the left (27,31). An important conclusion from these data is that a differential white count should be performed.

Other age changes include skin test changes and pain sensitivity. Changes in skin reactivity occur with age and may be related to prognosis (69). Silent pneumonia occurs in some 20 percent without pain. Silent myocardial infarctions are already well-characterized, but this also applies to the elderly with pneumonia.

Differential Diagnosis

One has to rule out cancer by bronchoscopy in selected elderly patients: patients over age 50 (pneumonia limited to one lobe); patients with 40 or more pack years of smoking; and patients with incomplete resolution after three weeks of treatment (58). One also has to rule out tuberculosis. We have just completed an autopsy study in people at age 85 and older--four percent of these people died with active tuberculosis (81). Two percent of these were definitely known to have tuberculosis, but in two percent, it probably was not known. This is a significant number of individuals.

TREATMENT

Prevention

A high proportion of pneumonia- and influenza-associated deaths involve persons aged 65 and older (2), primarily because only about 20 percent of this target elderly population receive influenza vaccine. Influenza vaccine can reduce the incidence and severity of influenza infections and subsequent pneumonia, particularly in the chronically ill elderly in nursing homes. When 79 percent or more of residents are vaccinated, influenza incidence and subsequent cases of pneumonia have been reduced as much as threefold, despite somewhat lower titers than those found in younger adults.

Pneumococcal vaccine is recommended for all patients over age 50 with a high risk of serious infection, except for those with multiple myeloma or treated Hodgkin's disease. Elderly hospitalized patients should be evaluated carefully for the use of the vaccine, as 87 percent of patients seen with pneumococcal pneumonia have been hospitalized at least once in the previous three years (55). All high risk outpatients have also made at least one outpatient visit in the three years before the onset of their pneumococcal infection, when vaccine could have been administered. Vaccine types have been isolated from 74 percent of elderly patients with pneumococcal pneumonia (2,84) and 84 percent of patients with pneumococcal septicemia (88).

Antibiotic Kinetics

A study in nine nursing homes in Seattle, Washington, (done for a different purpose) showed that when febrile elderly were treated, the case fatality rate fell to about one-fifth to one-sixth of what it was when no antibiotics were used in patients with various locations of the infection (12). Therefore, antibiotic treatment is effective in the elderly. You cannot intelligently treat "lobar" pneumonia and you cannot treat "bronchial" pneumonia, but you can treat pneumococcal pneumonia and you can treat Legionella or gram-negative rod pneumonia. A bacterial etiology must be determined; this is often missed in nursing home studies. It is very important to avoid taking these patients out of the mainstream of medicine. One must make sure that the laboratory tests they need are available and, thereby, make sure that they get the proper kind of treatment.

We do not have adequate data for all antibiotics. However, ceftazidime has been studied in the young and the old (Ref. 52 and Table 5). Studies must be done in normal young against normal elderly, and also in infected young against infected elderly. We did a study (77) in which we took the FDA original protocols for studying cephalothin and restudied the differences in the young and old. This can and should be done with many other antibiotics.

A randomized study of anaerobic pulmonary infections (primarily aspiration pneumonia) compared metronidazole and clindamycin treatment (55). There is an inadequate number of other studies comparing one antibiotic with another in the elderly. It is very important for such studies to be conducted.

Treatment of the Gram-Negative Pneumonia

Gram-negative pneumonia is usually hospital- or nursing home-acquired. The treatment frequently requires an aminoglycoside antibiotic, such as gentamicin, tobramycin, or amikacin, with or without penicillin or cephalosporin (71).

The aminoglycosides are known for their nephrotoxicities and ototoxicities, problems of heightened concern in the elderly, secondary to the reduced renal function that accompanies aging (16). This decline in renal function is not necessarily a contraindication to the use of aminoglycosides in the elderly. Several methods for dosing aminoglycosides have been proposed (15,18,72). Each of these methods gives a loading dose followed by a maintenance dose, based on the patient's estimated creatinine clearance, and requires the monitoring of aminoglycoside serum concentrations. Cockcroft and Gault (16) developed an equation that estimates an adult male's creatinine clearance from the patient's serum creatinine:

$$\frac{(140 - \text{Age in Years})(\text{Ideal Body Weight in Kg})}{72 \times \text{serum creatinine (mg/100 ml)}}$$

Multiplying this value by 0.85 approximates creatinine clearance for adult women. Peak (one-hour postinfusion) and trough (just prior to the next dose) serum concentrations should be drawn after the patient has reached a steady-state on an initial maintenance dose. The time required to be within ten percent of the average steady-state concentration is equal to four times the biologic half-life of a given drug, provided a loading dose was not given (33). Some practitioners choose to draw serum levels after the fifth dose; however, their patients may not necessarily be at steady-state, since the aminoglycoside half-lives are a function of renal activity, with half-lives ranging from 3.1 to 20.4 hours for persons with a creatinine clearance of 90 ml/min or 10 ml/min, respectively (72). Dosage adjustments can then be made by either increasing or decreasing the dose, or by lengthening or shortening the dosing interval.

It is generally felt that peak gentamicin and tobramycin levels should be less than 12 mcg/ml in order to decrease the risk of nephrotoxicity and ototoxicity (28). Amikacin's peaks should be below 32 to 34 mcg/ml (37). These values have been challenged, since these levels were obtained after serum creatinine had increased, and therefore, nephrotoxicity had already occurred (45).

Trough levels have also been implicated in association with nephrotoxicity, with troughs greater than 2 mcg/ml (for gentamicin and tobramycin) reported to be a risk factor (19,38). For amikacin, troughs greater than 10 mcg/ml have been implicated to increase the risk of toxicity (17). Again, similar controversy exists regarding the ability of trough concentrations to predict nephrotoxicity for the same reasons previously discussed in regard to peak levels (45,61).

On the other hand, peak and trough levels have been associated with efficacy. Moore et al. (60) analyzed the results of four prospective, randomized, double-blind, controlled trials of patients treated for gram-negative pneumonia with an aminoglycoside. Their results indicated a greater success rate (78 vs 22 percent) when peak serum concentrations were ≥ 7 mcg/ml for gentamicin and tobramycin, and ≥ 28 mcg/ml for amikacin. No difference in the incidence of nephrotoxicity was found.

Recent advances in antibiotic therapy offer the second and third generation cephalosporins as therapeutic alternatives for the treatment of pneumonia (6,7,13,34,39,50,56,76). Few, if any, adequately controlled comparison studies have been conducted between cephalosporin and the more traditional antimicrobial regimens in the management of pneumonia in elderly patients. Few cephalosporins have been studied from a pharmacokinetic standpoint in comparison of young subjects vs the elderly (Table 5, Ref. 52). We feel this type of information is important and useful, and we encourage such studies for all drugs used in the elderly.

TABLE 5. Pharmacokinetics of ceftazidime[a]

	Young	Old
Creatinine clearance	101	79[b]
Half-life clearance	1.89	2.72[b]
Area under curve	277	394
Volume of distribution	18	22[b]
Total clearance	110	88[b]
Renal clearance	82	69
Urinary recovery in 12 hours	87	75

[a]Adapted from Reference 52
[b]$p < .01$

Treatment of Gram-Positive Pneumonia

Rozas and Goldman (71) outlined a therapeutic regimen for the management of gram-positive pneumonia in the elderly. In previously healthy outpatients with a gram-positive pneumonia, based on gram-stained sputum samples, an administration of penicillin G (300,000 to 1,000,000 units i.v. every four to six hours) or penicillin V potassium (500 mg po every six hours) should be initiated. Patients with a penicillin allergy should be started on erythromycin, 250-500 mg po or i.v. every six hours (30,35,59). Similar treatment regimens are recommended for patients unable to produce a sputum sample. Patients with a postinfluenzal, hospital-acquired gram-positive pneumonia, or chronically ill outpatients (diabetes mellitus, COPD, uremia, ethanol abuse, etc.) with a gram-positive pneumonia should receive a penicillinase-resistant penicillin such as oxacillin, 1-2 grams i.v. every four to six hours (8).

Treatment of Other Pneumonias

Anaerobic pneumonias are a concern in the elderly, due to the increased incidence of aspiration pneumonias (3,91). Bartlett and Gorbach (4) studied 84 patients with a diagnosis of anaerobic aspiration pneumonitis or lung abscess. Forty-nine patients were treated with parenteral penicillin G, 1.8 to 10 million units/day for at least three days, followed by oral penicillin therapy, and 35 patients were treated with parenteral clindamycin, 900-1800 mg/day, followed by oral clindamycin therapy. No difference was found between the two groups in terms of time required to become afebrile, clearing by x-ray, and ultimate outcome. Two patients in the penicillin-treated group died of infection. There were no deaths due to infection in the clindamycin-treated group. There was no difference between the two groups in response by patients infected with __Bacteroides fragilis__. The authors concluded that penicillin G is the drug of choice for pulmonary infections involving anaerobic bacteria, and that clindamycin is an alternate choice when penicillin G is contraindicated. This study has been criticized because the authors do not mention randomization or blinding (5).

Levison et al. (51) in a randomized study, compared the efficacy of penicillin G, one million units i.v. every four hours, to anaerobic lung infections (41,74). Patients were changed to similar oral therapy following clinical improvement. Patients treated with clindamycin became afebrile sooner and had fewer days of fetid sputum. Four of the 20 patients treated with penicillin had significant extensions of their infection. Of those patients available for followup, eight of the 15 patients treated with penicillin were cured four weeks after discontinuation of therapy; all 13 patients in the clindamycin-treated group were cured. The authors concluded that pencillin may not be the optimal therapy for anaerobic lung abscess. Metronidazole does not appear to be an alternative to clindamycin in anaerobic pulmonary infections (67).

Drug-resistant (ampicillin and, rarely, chloramphenicol) Hemophilus influenzae pneumonia in the elderly (36,83) has been reported in up to 25 percent of cases. Bronchitis and harmless pharyngeal carriage can also occur, but this organism can be the second-most common cause of pneumonia in the elderly. Cough and sputum production with fever, chills, shortness of breath, and vague chest pain occur. Pleural effusion may coexist. It is important to get an adequate sputum specimen using chest percussion, ultrasonic nebulizers, and sometimes transtracheal aspiration. Culture on chocolate agar is necessary. Treatment is with chloramphenicol or cefamandole.

Postoperative pneumonia (57) occurs in only one to two percent of all operative cases (but more frequently in the elderly); however, it comprises ten percent of all fatal postoperative cases. It is most often found in emergency operations; is postatelectatic; is respirator-associated; is associated with fluid overload; or is postoperative with peritonitis. It is usually gram-negative in type.

Superinfections (73) causing pneumonia, are found in several different conditions: Hodgkin's disease; leukocyte defects; underlying disease plus steroid or antibiotics; pneumonias secondary to operations or procedures such as endotracheal intubation or respirator use; infections due to overuse of inappropriate antibiotics; and in elderly patients with alcohol or drug abuse. Recurrent pneumonia (48) in the elderly can occur with emphysema, congestive heart failure, bronchiectasis, previous pulmonary tuberculosis, previous lung resection, bronchial cancer, with esophageal disorders such as Zenker's diverticulum, and with systemic diseases such as chronic alcoholism, diabetes mellitus, chronic sinusitis, and epilepsy. Chronic steroid therapy can also lead to recurrent pneumonia.

Intracellular Penetration of Antibiotics

It must be recognized that an antibiotic is of little value if it does not reach the parasite causing the infection. Some parasites occur within the polymorphonuclear leukocyte (68) or within the macrophages (44,46), e.g., <u>Staphylococcus aureus</u>, Salmonella, Listeria, Legionella, tubercle bacilli, and Brucella. They are not very common, but <u>S. aureus</u> can be very lethal in the elderly and Legionella is not uncommon. Therefore, we have to pay attention to which antibiotics penetrate intracellularly. For example, clindamycin and erythromycin penetrate intracellularly very well, and some of the other drugs do it quite poorly (68). The passage of the antibiotic from the serum into the bronchus is very important (1,10,11,14,21,63-66,75). We found in our study of cephalothin in the aged that they responded very poorly compared to the young when treated for pneumonia (77), although other infections in the elderly responded well to cephalothin. One of the reasons for the poor response in pneumonia in the elderly may be poor penetration. Antibiotics that get into the sputum well are minocycline, gentamicin, amikacin, tobramycin, and clindamycin (63). Lung tissue concentrations of antibiotics have seldom been measured (87,90). Some studies are available but they are not necessarily differentiated into young and old people, nor into noninfected and infected patients, and many have been performed in canines. Further studies are needed, especially those focusing on the elderly.

PROGNOSIS

Can we identify those people who are in danger of dying and if so, what can we do about it (23)? Empyema may contain 1,700 cc of pus in an elderly patient. If each cc of this material contains 10^5 bacteria or more, and the 1,700 cc is 10^3 in logarithms, that is 10^8 that the physician can aspirate from the chest, using a syringe or chest tube. Experimental data on animals can be extrapolated to 60 kg people, suggesting that it takes 10^{13} bacteria to kill a person. If you can remove 10^8 organisms which increase by one logarithm hourly, you are taking the patient away from the point of death much more quickly than any antibiotic treatment. Draining an empyema or draining an abscess, therefore, is very important. Other indications of severity would be a spread to some tissue such as a joint or the central nervous system or the presence of a positive blood culture.

How do we measure prognosis in the elderly? One must first consider the nature of the insult, that is, the type of invading organism. In all age groups, Pseudomonas pneumonia is very much more lethal than pneumococcal pneumonia. What is the quantity of the insult: one lobe <u>vs</u> two lobes, negative blood cultures <u>vs</u> positive blood cultures? What underlying host diseases are present in elderly people, and how many complications? A study from Johns Hopkins (85) shows untreated pneumococcal pneumonia compared to treated pneumococcal pneumonia. Overall, five percent was the case fatality rate with penicillin treatment compared to 30 percent without antibiotic. In the young (10 to 20 years of age), one percent compared to ten percent untreated; in the old (age 60 and over), eight percent compared to 72 percent, when treated and untreated cases are compared. One lobe involvement is significantly different in case fatality rates compared to two lobes.

Underlying disease is significant in increasing the case fatality rate and the presence of positive blood cultures is also significant. Many of these problems occur in pneumonia in the elderly. What is needed is a prognostic score which can be made on admission of a patient to the hospital similar to that used in meningitis.

CONCLUSION

Pneumonia is a very significant illness in the elderly. It is causing unnecessary deaths in many elderly persons, more in males than in females. Pneumonia may partially explain the differential survival rate in men and women. There is a very significant difference in the quantity (85 vs 50 percent) of serious underlying disease in elderly people with pneumonia which has to receive treatment at the same time as pneumonia. If these factors are attended to and a proper diagnosis is made with culture and sensitivities of the causative agent, then the elderly are very treatable. If we do treat them, many should survive (78). Continued studies of antibiotic kinetics in normal and infected elderly, as well as basic studies in experimental pneumonias (26) are essential if the high toll of pneumonia-related deaths in the elderly is to be reduced.

REFERENCES

1. Alexander, M.R., Schoell, J., Hicklin, C., Kasik, J.E., and Coleman, D. (1982): Am. Rev. Respir. Dis., 125:208-209.
2. Barker, W.H., and Mullooly, J.P. (1982): Arch. Intern. Med., 142:85-89.
3. Bartlett, J.G., and Gorbach, S.L. (1975): Chest, 68:560-566.
4. Bartlett, J.G., and Gorbach, S.L. (1975): JAMA, 234:935-937.
5. Bartlett, J.G., Gorbach, S.L., and Finegold, S.M. (1974): Am. J. Med., 56:202-207.
6. Baumgartner, J.D., and Glauser, M.P. (1984): Am. J. Med., 66:54-58.
7. Bentley, D.W. (1984): Gerontology, 30:297-307.

8. Berk, S.L., Gallemore, G.M., and Smith, J.K. (1981): J. Am. Geriatr. Soc., 29:319-321.
9. Berk, S.L., Holtsclaw, S.A., Wiener, S.L., and Smith, J.K. (1982): Arch. Intern. Med., 142:537-539.
10. Berk, S.L., Neumann, P., Holtsclaw, S., and Smith, J.K. (1982): Am. J. Med., 72:899-902.
11. Braude, A.C., Hornstein, A., Klein, M., Vas, A., and Rebuck, A.S. (1983): Am. Rev. Respir. Dis., 127:563-565.
12. Brown, N.K., and Thompson, D.J. (1979): N. Engl. J. Med., 300:1246-1250.
13. Castleton, B., Goodwin, C.S., Stirling, J., Pitcher-Wilmott, R., and Elton, S. (1976): Age Ageing, 5:181-187.
14. Casto, D.T., Gal, P., McCue, J.D., and Zumwalt, A.A. (1985): Clin. Pharm., 4:67-70.
15. Chan, R.A., Benner, E.J., and Hoeprich, R.D. (1978): Ann. Intern. Med., 76:775-778.
16. Cockcroft, D.W., and Gault, M.H. (1976): Nephron, 16:31-41.
17. Darwin, E.Z. (1980) In: Applied Pharmacokinetics: Principles of Therapeutic Drug Monitoring, edited by W.E. Evans, J.J. Schentag, and W.J. Jusko, pp. 210-239. Applied Therapeutics, Inc., San Francisco, California.
18. Dettle, I.C. (1974): Clin. Pharmacol. Ther., 16:274-280.
19. Dohlgren, J.G., Anderson, E.T., and Hewitt, W.L. (1975): Antimicrob. Agents Chemother., 8:58-62.
20. Dorff, G.J., Rytel, M.W., Farmer, S.G., and Scanlon, G. (1973): Am. J. Med. Sci., 255:349-358.
21. Dull, W.L., Alexander, M.R., and Kasik, J.E. (1979): Antimicrob. Agents Chemother., 16:767-771.
22. Ebright, J.R., and Rytel, M.W. (1980): J. Am. Geriatr. Soc., 28:220.
23. Editorial (1983): J. Infect. Dis., January, 20.
24. Ellenbogen, C., Graybill, J.R., Sliva, J., and Homme, P.J. (1974): Am. J. Med., 56:169-177.
25. Esposito, A.L. (1984): Arch. Intern. Med., 144:945-948.
26. Esposito, A.L., and Pennington, J.E. (1983): Am. Rev. Respir. Dis., 128:662-667.
27. Everett, E.D., Rahm, A.E., Jr., Adoniya, R., Stevens, D.L., and McNitt, T.R. (1977): JAMA, 238:319-321.
28. Falco, F.G., Smith, H.M., and Arcieri, G.M. (1969): J. Infect. Dis., 119:406-409.
29. Fedson, D.S., and Baldwin, J.A. (1982): JAMA, 248:1989-1995.
30. Fraschini, F., Braga, P.C., Copponi, V., Maccari, M., Piovania, D., Scaglione, F., and Scarpazza, G. (1981): Curr. Med. Res. Opin., 7:429-439.
31. Gabbert, W., Hutaff, L.W., and Harrell, G.T. (1974): Geriatrics, 29:96-100.
32. Garb, J.L., Brown, R.B., Garb, J.R., and Tuthill, R.W. (1978): JAMA, 240:2169-2172.

33. Gibaldi, M., and Pevier, D. (1982): Pharmacokinetics. Marcel Dekker, Inc., New York.
34. Gleckman, R.A., and Esposito, A.L. (1979): J. Am. Geriatr. Soc., 27:345-347.
35. Gleckman, R.A., and Roth, R.M. (1984): Pharmacotherapy, 4:81-88.
36. Gleckman, R.A., and Roth, R.M. (1984): Geriatrics, 39: 51-53, 56-58, 60.
37. Gooding, P.G., Berman, E., Lane, A.Z., and Agre, K. (1976): J. Infect. Dis., 134:S441-S445.
38. Goodman, E.L., Van Gelder, J., Holmes, R., Hull, A.R., and Sanford, J.P. (1975): Antimicrob. Agents Chemother., 8:434-438.
39. Grieco, M.M., Lange, M., Daniels, J.A., Den, M., Amaram, N., and Kornfeld, H. (1982): J. Antimicrob. Chemother., 10 (Suppl. C):223-225.
40. Haleem, M.A. (1982): Gerontology, 28:203-207.
41. Hand, W.L., and King-Thompson, N.L. (1982): Antimicrob. Agents Chemother., 21:241-247.
42. Heffron, R. (1939, reprinted 1979): Pneumonia. Harvard University Press, Boston, Massachusetts.
43. Helms, C.M. (1980): Geriatrics, 35:87-94.
44. Hill, C.D., and Stamm, W.E. (1982): Geriatrics, 37:40-50.
45. Jerome, J.S. (1980): In: Applied Pharmacokinetics: Principles of Therapeutic Drug Monitoring, edited by W.E. Evans, J.J. Schentag, and W.J. Jusko, pp. 174-209. Applied Therapeutics, Inc., San Francisco, California.
46. Johnson, J.D., Hand, W.L., Francis, J.B., King-Thompson, N. and Corwin, R.W. (1980): J. Lab. Clin. Med., 95:429-439.
47. Kannel, W.B. (1982): In: Biological Markers of Aging, edited by M.E. Reff and E.L. Schneider, NIH Publication 82-2221, USDHHS, Washington, D.C.
48. Khokhar, N. (1983): Hosp. Pract., 18:157-158.
49. Kneeland, Y., Jr., and Price, K.M. (1960): Am. J. Med., 29:967-979.
50. Lee, G.S., Kakati, R., and Mahmoud, I.A. (1980): Curr. Med. Res. Opin., 6:564-568.
51. Levison, M.E., Mangura, C.T., Lorber, B., Abrutyn, E., Pesanti, E.L., Levy, R.S., MacGregor, R.R., and Schwartz, A.R. (1983): Ann. Intern. Med., 98:466-471.
52. Ljungberg, B., and Nilsson-Ehle, I. (1984): Scand. J. Infect. Dis., 16:325-326.
53. Macfarlane, J.T., Finch, R.G., Ward, M.J., and Macrae, A.D. (1982): Lancet ii:255-258.
54. Macfarlane, J.T., Finch, R.G., Ward, M.J., and Rose, D.H. (1983): J. Infect., 7:111-117.
55. Magnussen, C.T., and Valenti, W.M. (1984): Arch. Intern. Med., 144:1755-1757.
56. Mandell, G.L. (1980): Scand. J. Infect. Dis., 25 (Suppl.): 107-111.

57. Martin, L.G., Asher, E.F., Casey, J.M., and Fry, D.E. (1984): Arch. Surg., 119:379-383.
58. McDowell, D.E. (1980): South. Med. J., 73:761-762.
59. Middleton, R.S.W. (1974): Gerontol. Clin. (Basel), 16:92-99.
60. Moore, R.D., Smith, C.R., and Lietman, P.S. (1984): Am. J. Med., 77:657-662.
61. Moore, R.D., Smith, C.R., Lipsky, J.J., Mellits, E.D., and Lietman, P.S. (1984): Ann. Intern. Med., 100:352-357.
62. Mrazek, S.W. (1969): J. Am. Geriatr. Soc., 17:969-973.
63. Pennington, J.E. (1981): Rev. Infect. Dis., 3:67-73.
64. Pennington, J.E., and Reynolds, H.Y. (1973): J. Infect. Dis., 128:63-68.
65. Pennington, J.E., and Reynolds, H.Y. (1975): J. Infect. Dis., 131:158-162.
66. Pennington, J.E., Reynolds, H.Y., Dale, D.C., and MacLowry, J.D. (1975): J. Infect. Dis., 132:270-275.
67. Perlino, C.A. (1981): Arch. Intern. Med., 141:1424-1427.
68. Prokesch, R.C., and Hand, W.L. (1982): Antimicrob. Agents Chemother., 21:373-380.
69. Roberts-Thompson, I.C., Whittingham, S., Youngchaiyud, U., and Mackay, I.R. (1974): Lancet ii:368-370.
70. Roth, R.M., and Gleckman, R.A. (1985): Am. Fam. Physician, 31:131-137.
71. Rozas, C.J., and Goldman, A.L. (1982): Geriatrics, 37:61-66.
72. Sarubbi, F.A., and Hull, J.H. (1978): Ann. Intern. Med., 89:612-618.
73. Sen, P., Kapila, R., Chmel, H., Armstrong, D.A., and Louria, D.B. (1982): Am. J. Med., 73:706-718.
74. Sen, P., Tecson, F., Kapila, R., and Louria, D.B. (1974): Arch. Intern. Med., 134:73-77.
75. Smith, B.R., and Lefrock, J.L. (1983): Chest, 83:904-908.
76. Smith, C.R., Ambinder, R., Lipsky, J.J., Petty, B.G., Israel, E., Levitt, R., Mellits, E.D., Rocco, L., Longstreth, J., and Lietman, P.S. (1984): Ann. Intern. Med., 101:469-477.
77. Smith, I.M. (1971): Postgrad. Med. J., 47 (Suppl.):78-87.
78. Smith, I.M. (1982): Hosp. Pract., 17:69-77, 81-85.
79. Smith, I.M. (1985): In: Relations Between Normal Aging and Disease, edited by H.A. Johnson, pp. 101-115. Raven Press, New York.
80. Smith, I.M. (1986): Manuscript in preparation.
81. Smith, I.M., and Lorkovic (1986): Manuscript in preparation.
82. Smith, I.M., and Smith, J.M. (1984): In: Immunology and Infection in the Elderly, edited by R.A. Fox, pp. 21-43. Churchill Livingstone, Edinburgh.
83. Stratton, C.W., Hawley, H.B., Horsman, T.A., Tu, K.K., Ackley, A., Fernando, N.K., and Weinstein, M.P. (1980): Am. Rev. Respir. Dis., 121:595-598.

84. Valenti, W.M., Jenzer, M., and Bentley, D.W. (1978): Am. Rev. Respir. Dis., 117:233-238.
85. Van Meter, Jr., T.E. (1954): N. Engl. J. Med., 251:1048-1052.
86. Verghese, A., and Berk, S.L. (1983): Medicine, 62:271-284.
87. Wartenberg, K., Tonak, J., and Knapp, W. (1983): Infection, 11:280-282.
88. Weisholtz, S.J., Hartman, B.J., and Roberts, R.B. (1983): Am. J. Med., 77:199-204.
89. Wolk, P.J., and Apicella, M.A. (1978): Arch. Intern. Med., 138:1084-1085.
90. Wollmer, P., Pride, N.B., Rhodes, C.G., Sanders, A., Pike, V.W., Palmer, A.J., Silvester, D.J., and Liss, R.H. (1982): Lancet ii:1361-1364.
91. Zavala, D.C. (1977): Geriatrics, 32:46-51.
92. Ziskind, M.M., Schwarz, M.I., George, R.B., Weill, H., Shames, J.M., Herbert, S.J., and Ichinose, H. (1970): Ann. Intern. Med., 72:835-839.

EFFECT OF AGE ON THE IMMUNOLOGICAL DEFENSE SYSTEM:
THE GENETIC EXPRESSION OF SPECIFIC AND NONSPECIFIC MEDIATORS

Arlan Richardson,* Wutong Wu,[†] Mark S. Rutherford,***
Dian-dong Li,[††] Mohammad A. Pahlavani,** and H. Tak Cheung**

Departments of *Chemistry and **Biological Sciences,
Illinois State University, Normal, Illinois 61761;
***Department of Veterinary Pathobiology,
University of Illinois, Urbana, Illinois 61801; and
[†]Department of Biochemistry, Nanjing College of Pharmacy and
[††]Institute of Antibiotics, Chinese Academy of Medical Sciences,
The People's Republic of China

Gene expression is a fundamental process that occurs in all living cells and plays a basic role in the mechanisms involved in an organism adapting to a variety of stimuli. During the past two decades, many investigators have compared the translational and transcriptional activities of tissues from young and old organisms (for a review see references 17-20). In general, the data from these studies have shown that a decline in both of these processes occurs with increasing age. In fact, because most organisms and tissues show an age-related decline in protein synthesis, Richardson and Cheung (23) suggested that the decline in protein synthesis might be an important factor in the mechanism underlying the aging process.

Although the effect of aging on gene expression has been studied extensively in a variety of tissues, there is very little information on how changes in gene expression could affect the immune system. This is ironic in light of the fact that the immune response of an organism declines dramatically with increasing age (16,35). An age-related decline in gene expression could have important consequences in the immunological defense of an organism because the initiation of the immune response after antigenic stimulation depends on the synthesis of a diverse array of protein mediators that have both effector and regulatory functions (28,40). The cascade of immunological events also depends on the expression of appropriate receptors on the surface of cells that will eventually carry out specific immune functions (1,15). There is direct evidence for the requirement of protein synthesis and RNA synthesis in the immune system. The production of lymphokines, e.g., interleukin 2 (9,38), interleukin 3 (17), macrophage activator factor (32,33), chemotactic factors (32,33), and monokines, such as interleukin 1 (2), depends on the synthesis of mRNA. Inhibitors of RNA synthesis will abrogate the production of these lymphokines and result in the termination of the immune response (32,33). Furthermore, the expression of interleukin 2 receptors, which are crucial in the proliferative response to antigenic challenge, also depends on the synthesis of mRNA (20,29). Therefore, it is obvious that any defect in the ability of cells to express a particular protein could lead to an impairment of the immune response.

In 1983, we suggested that a decrease in gene expression might play a role in the age-related decline in the immune system (5). As shown in Fig. 1A, we found that the protein synthetic activity of mitogen-stimulated lymphocytes from rat spleen declined significantly with increasing age. The decline in protein synthesis paralleled the decline in mitogen-induced lymphocyte proliferation. More recently, Tollefsbol and Cohen (31) confirmed our studies with lymphocytes from human subjects. As shown in Fig. 1B, the incorporation of leucine

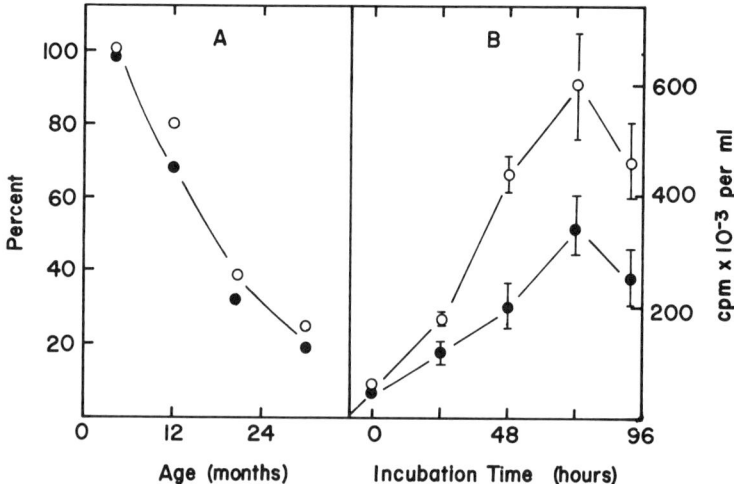

FIG. 1. The effect of age on protein synthesis by lymphocytes. The data in Fig. 1A were taken from Cheung et al. (5) and show the incorporation of valine (o) into protein and lymphocyte proliferation (●) by concanavalin A-stimulated lymphocytes isolated from the spleen of male Fischer F344 rats. The data in Fig. 1B were taken from Tollefsbol and Cohen (31) and show the incorporation of leucine by phytohemagglutinin-stimulated lymphocytes from young (o) and elderly (●) human subjects.

into protein by mitogen-stimulated lymphocytes from young (23 to 32 years) subjects was higher than that of lymphocytes from elderly (70 to 80 years) subjects.

Because our initial studies indicated that a decline in translation occurred with age in lymphoid tissue, our laboratories have studied the expression of specific genes that act as rather specific or nonspecific mediators in the immune system.

SPECIFIC MEDIATORS (THE INTERLEUKINS)

Most immune mediators are produced by either lymphocytes or macrophages and are required in the development and generation of specific immune responses. The interleukins are the most studied of the specific mediators and play critical roles in clonal expansion, inactivation, and differentiation of effector and regulatory immunocytes. One of the first interleukins to be identified and studied was interleukin 2 (IL 2). The early studies by Morgan et al. (18) showed that conditioned media from mitogen-stimulated lymphocyte cultures promoted the long term proliferation of cloned T cells. The factor responsible for this activity was initially called T cell growth factor. Using cloned T cell proliferation as an assay, it was possible to purify and characterize IL 2. IL 2 is a 15,000 to 22,000 dalton glycoprotein that is produced by T cells in response to stimulation by antigens and lectins in the presence of adherent cells (7,36). IL 2 has been shown to be essential for mitogenesis. The binding of IL 2 to IL 2 receptors on the surface of responding T cells drives the cells into proliferation. In addition to being required for the proliferation of T cells, IL 2 enhances thymocyte proliferation (27) and induces cytotoxic T cell activation in cultures of mouse cells (34). Because IL 2 is a key immunoregulator, changes in IL 2 expression could be an important factor in the age-related change in the immunological status of an organism.

Recently, several laboratories, including our laboratories, showed that the production of IL 2 declined with increasing age (4,5,10,30). We found that the decline in IL 2 paralleled the decline in mitogen-induced lymphocyte proliferation observed in Fig. 1A. Using a monoclonal antibody to IL 2 and a cDNA probe to IL 2, we have measured the genetic expression of IL 2 at the levels of translation and transcription. As shown in Fig. 2, the levels of IL 2 in the culture supernatants of mitogen-induced lymphocytes decreased 74 percent between 5 and 23 months of age. This decrease is similar to the decrease in IL 2 levels that has been reported previously (5). The polypeptides in the culture supernatants were concentrated and resolved by gel electrophoresis, and the IL 2 was identified by Western Blot Analysis using the monoclonal antibody to IL 2. There was no apparent age-related change in the size of the IL 2 (data not shown).

The synthesis of IL 2 was measured as the incorporation of radioactive valine into material precipitated by a monoclonal antibody to IL 2. As shown in Fig. 2, the synthesis of IL 2 declined 65 percent with increasing age. The decline in IL 2 synthesis and IL 2 activity was identical. Therefore, the decline in IL 2 levels, which had been reported previously, is due to decreased IL 2 synthesis and is not due to a rapid utilization or destruction of IL 2.

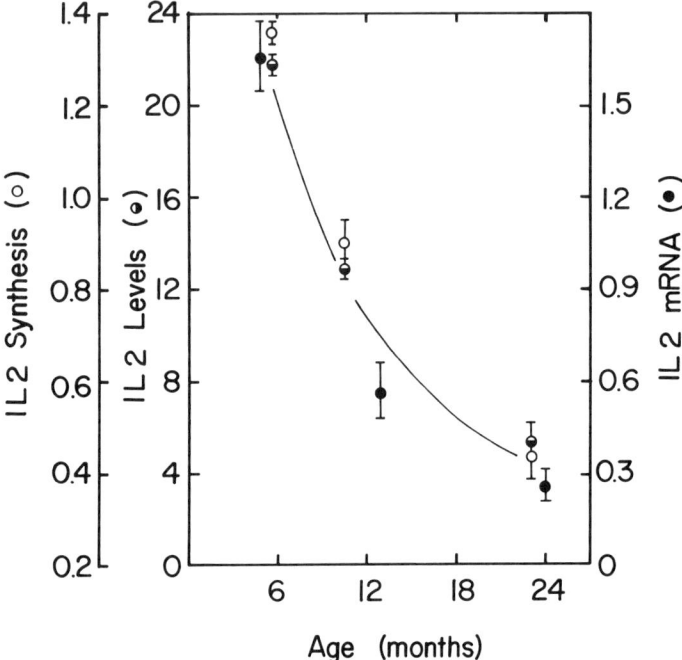

FIG. 2. The effect of age on the genetic expression of IL 2. Lymphocytes isolated from the spleens of male Fischer F344 rats were stimulated with concanavalin A (5 µg/ml) for 20 hours and the expression of IL 2 was measured. The levels of IL 2 (units/ml) were measured by the ability of the culture supernatants to support the growth of cloned T cells; the synthesis of IL 2 (pmoles of valine/min/10^7 cells) was measured by the amount of radioactive valine incorporated into material precipitated by the monoclonal antibody to IL 2; and the levels of IL 2 mRNA (area) were measured by cytoplasmic dot blot hybridization (39).

The levels of IL 2 mRNA in mitogen-stimulated lymphocytes was measured by hybridization using a cDNA probe to IL 2 (39). As shown in Fig. 2, the levels of IL 2 mRNA induced by concanavalin A decreased 78 percent between 5 and 24 months of age. The decrease in IL 2 mRNA was not due to an age-related increase in mRNA degradation (data not shown). Thus, the data in Fig. 2 clearly show that the age-related decline in IL 2 production by mitogen-stimulated lymphocytes is due to a decrease in the genetic expression of IL 2.

Recently, we have turned our attention to the effect of age on the expression of interleukin 3 (IL 3). IL 3 is produced by mitogen- or antigen-stimulated T cells and is involved in the regulation of the growth and differentiation of pluripotent stem cells. A broad range of biological activities have been ascribed to IL 3, e.g., multicolony stimulating factor (3), hematopoietic growth factor (3), burst promoting activity (13), P cell stimulating factor (26), mast cell growth factor (19), histamine producing cell stimulating factor (8), and thy-1-inducing activity (12,19). IL 3 is a glycosylated protein of 28,000 to 32,500 daltons (3,11). The expression of IL 2 and IL 3 was measured concomitantly in mitogen-stimulated lymphocytes from mice using cDNA probes to IL 2 and IL 3. As shown previously for lymphocytes from rats (Fig. 2), a decline in IL 2 levels was observed with increasing age. In addition,

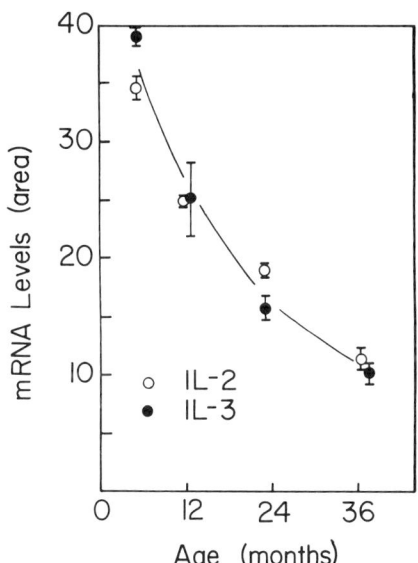

FIG. 3. The effect of age on the expression of IL 2 and IL 3. Lymphocytes isolated from the spleens of 5- to 37-month-old male C57Bl/6J mice were cultured with concanavalin A (5 μg/ml) for 20 hours. The levels of IL 2 and IL 3 mRNA induced by concanavalin A were determined by cytoplasmic dot blot hybridization (39). The amount of the cDNA probe that hybridized to the dot blots was quantified by autoradiography and is presented as the area of the densitometer scans.

Fig. 3 shows that the levels of IL 3 induced by concanavalin A decreased 74 percent between 5 and 37 months of age. Therefore, a dramatic age-related decline in the induction of two interleukins, IL 2 and IL 3, was observed in mitogen-stimulated lymphocytes.

NONSPECIFIC MEDIATORS (THE COMPLEMENT FACTORS)

The complement system comprises a group of proteins that carry out nonspecific immunological functions. These include the complement factors of the classical and alternative pathways which lead to the production of activated polypeptides. These activated factors have diverse, nonspecific immunological activities. The ultimate result of complement activation is the disruption of biological membranes of gram negative bacteria which results in cell lysis. The complement system is also important in binding, internalizing, and degrading immune complexes (14); and it stimulates the release of regulatory mediators by macrophages and mast cells (25). Most of the proteins of the complement system are produced by cells of nonlymphoid tissues, e.g., hepatocytes and fibroblasts (6).

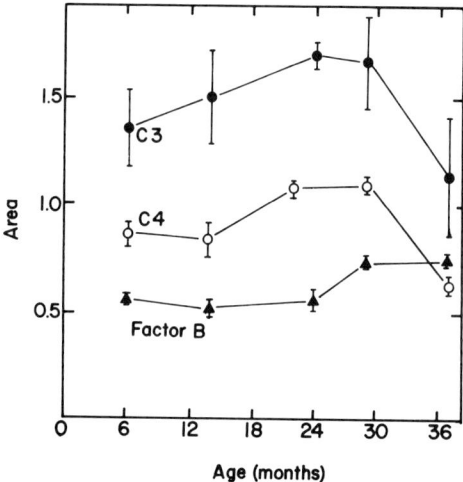

FIG. 4. The effect of age on the expression of complement factors by the liver. RNA was isolated from 5- to 37-month-old male Fischer F344 rats. The levels of C3, C4, and factor B were measured by dot blot hybridization (37). The amount of the cDNA probe that hybridized to the RNA was measured by autoradiography as is expressed as the area of the densitometer scans.

Because the liver plays an important role in the synthesis of several complement proteins and because it is well-documented that the translational (21,24) and transcriptional (22,24) activities of the liver decline with increasing age, we measured the levels of several genes that code for complement proteins, e.g., complement C3 (C3), complement C4 (C4), and complement protein factor B (factor B). C3 is the central complement protein in both the classical and alternative pathways. It is the most abundant of the complement proteins and it is primarily produced by the liver, as is factor B (6). C4 is a component of the classical pathway and is produced by hepatocytes and macrophages while factor B is a component of the alternative pathway.

The relative levels of C3, C4, and factor B in RNA isolated from the liver of rats are given in Fig. 4. The levels of these three mRNA species increased slightly (28 to 32 percent) between 5 and 29 months of age. The relative levels of C3 and C4 decreased between 29 and 37 months of age; however, the decrease in C3 was not statistically significant. In contrast, the level of factor B mRNA in 37-month-old rats remained significantly higher than that of 5-month-old rats.

DISCUSSION

The decline in the immune system is believed to be an important factor in the increased incidence of disease and cancer that is associated with age (16,35). One common assay for the immunological status of an organism is the ability of mitogens to induce lymphocyte proliferation. Although it is well-documented that the mitogen-induction of lymphocyte proliferation declines markedly with age, our current understanding of the biochemical mechanism underlying the decline in mitogenesis is very limited. The results of our research indicate that the age-related decrease in the appearance of IL 2 in culture supernatants is due to a decrease in the expression of the IL 2 gene; a decrease in the synthesis of IL 2 and the level of IL 2 mRNA paralleled the decrease in the level of IL 2 in the culture supernatants (Fig. 2). Because IL 2 plays a critical role in the response of T cells to mitogens, the decrease in the ability of T cells to express IL 2 could be an important factor in the age-related decline in mitogenesis and, also, the ability of the immune system to function.

Because a general decline in total protein synthesis is observed in mitogen-stimulated lymphocytes (Fig. 1), it is reasonable to assume that the expression of other genes by mitogen-stimulated lymphocytes is reduced with increasing age. Preliminary studies by our laboratory have shown that the mitogen-induction of IL 3 mRNA declines as a function of age (Fig. 3). This is the first evidence to show that the ability of lymphocytes to produce IL 3 declines with increasing age.

In contrast to lymphocytes, the liver showed no dramatic age-related change in the genetic expression of the three complement factors, e.g., C3, C4, and factor B. This observation is interesting because it is well-documented that total protein synthesis and total RNA synthesis declines with increasing age in the liver (21-24). Thus, our preliminary studies suggest that aging may have a greater effect on the expression of specific mediators by lymphocytes than the expression of nonspecific mediators by liver.

ACKNOWLEDGMENTS

This work was supported in part by grants AG 04520 and AG 04097 from the National Institute on Aging. We thank Dr. Kendall Smith of Dartmouth Medical School (Hanover, NH) for providing DMS anti-IL 2 producing hybridoma and to the following investigators for providing the cDNA clones used in this research: Dr. Tadatsugu Taniguchi of the Japanese Foundation for Cancer Research (Tokyo, Japan) for the cDNA probe to IL 2 mRNA from human; Dr. Frank Ruscetti of the Frederick Cancer Research Facility (Frederick, MD) for the cDNA probe to IL 2 from mouse; Dr. Ken-ichi Arai from DNAX Research Institute of Molecular and Cellular Biology (Palo Alto, CA) for the cDNA probe to IL 3 from mouse; Dr. George Fey of Scripps Clinic and Research Foundation (La Jolla, CA) for the cDNA probe to C3 from mouse liver; Dr. Masaru Nanaka of Kanazawa University (Kanazawa, Japan) for the cDNA probe to C4 from mouse liver; and Dr. R. Duncan Campbell of the University of Oxford (Oxford, United Kingdom) for the cDNA probe to factor B from human liver.

REFERENCES

1. Abo, T., Miller, C.A., Balch, C.M., and Cooper, M. (1983): J. Immunol., 131:1822-1826.
2. Auron, P.E., Webb, A.C., Rosenwasser, L.J., Mucci, S.F., Rich, A., Wolff, S.M., and Dinarrello, C. (1984): Proc. Natl. Acad. Sci. USA, 81:7907-7911.
3. Bazill, G.W., Haynes, M., Garland, J., and Dexter, T.M. (1983): Biochem. J., 210:747-759.
4. Chang, M.P., Makinodan, T., Peterson, W.J., and Strehler, B.L. (1982): J. Immunol., 129:2426-2430.
5. Cheung, H.T., Twu, J.S., and Richardson, A. (1983): Exp. Gerontol., 18:620-629.
6. Colten, H.R., and Einstein, L.P. (1976): Transplant. Rev., 32:3-25.
7. Di Sabato, G. (1982): Proc. Natl. Acad. Sci. USA, 79:3020-3023.
8. Dy, M., Lebel, B., Kamour, P., and Hamburger, J. (1981): J. Exp. Med., 153:293-309.

9. Elliott, J.F., Lin, Y., Minzel, S.B., Bleackley, R.C., Harnish, D.G., and Paetkau, V. (1984): Science, 226:1439-1441.
10. Gillis, S., Kozak, R., Durante, M., and Weksler, M.E. (1981): J. Clin. Invest., 67:937-942.
11. Ihle, J.N., Keller, J., Henderson, L., Klein, F., and Palaszynski, E. (1982): J. Immunol., 129:2431-2436.
12. Ihle, J.N., Keller, J., Oroszlan, S., Henderson, L.E., Copeland, T.D., Fitch, F., Prystowsky, M.B., Goldwasser, E., Schrader, J.W., Palaszynski, E., Dy, M., and Lebel, B. (1983): J. Immunol., 131:282-287.
13. Iscove, N.N., Roitsch, C.A., Williams, N., and Guilbert, L.L. (1982): J. Cell. Physiol. Suppl., 1:65-78.
14. Kijlstra, A., van Es, L.A., and Daha, M.R. (1981): Immunology, 43:345-352.
15. Lipkowitz, S., Greene, W., Rubin, A., Novogrodsky, A., and Stenzel, K. (1984): J. Immunol., 132:31-37.
16. Makinodan, T. (1978): Fed. Proc., 37:1239-1240.
17. Miyatake, S., Yokota, T., Lee, F., and Arai, K. (1985): Proc. Natl. Acad. Sci. USA, 82:316-320.
18. Morgan, D.A., Ruscetti, F.W., and Gallo, R.C. (1976): Science, 193:1007-1008.
19. Nabel, G., Galli, S.J., Dvorak, A.M., Dvorak, H.F., and Cantor, H. (1981): Nature, 291:332-334.
20. Reem, G., and Yeh, N. (1985): J. Immunol., 134:953-958.
21. Richardson, A., and Birchenall-Sparks, M.C. (1983): In: Review of Biological Research in Aging, Vol. 1, edited by M. Rothstein, pp. 255-273. Alan R. Liss, Inc., New York.
22. Richardson, A., Birchenall-Sparks, M.C., and Staecker, J.L. (1983): In: Review of Biological Research in Aging, Vol. 1, edited by M. Rothstein, pp. 275-294, Alan R. Liss, Inc., New York.
23. Richardson, A., and Cheung, H.T. (1982): Life Sci., 31:605-613.
24. Richardson, A., Roberts, M.S., and Rutherford, M.S. (1985): In: Review of Biological Research in Aging, Vol. 2, edited by M. Rothstein, pp. 395-419. Alan R. Liss, Inc., New York.
25. Rutherford, B., and Schenkein, H.A. (1983): J. Immunol., 130:874-877.
26. Schrader, J.W., Lewis, S.J., Clark-Lewis, I., and Culvenor, J.G. (1981): Proc. Natl. Acad. Sci. USA, 78:323-327.
27. Shaw, J., Monticone, V., and Paetkau, V. (1978): J. Immunol., 120:1967-1973.
28. Smith, K.A. (1984): In: Lymphokine Regulation of T Cell and B Cell Function, edited by W.E. Paul, pp. 559-576, Raven Press. New York.
29. Smith, K.A., and Cantrell, D.A. (1985): Proc. Natl. Acad. Sci. USA, 82:864-868.

30. Thoman, M., and Weigle, W. (1981): J. Immunol., 127:2102-2105.
31. Tollefsbol, T.D., and Cohen, H.J. (1985): Mech. Ageing Dev., 30:53-62.
32. Varesio, L., and Holden, H.T. (1980): J. Immunol., 124:2288-2294.
33. Varesio, L., Holden, H.T., and Tatamelli, D. (1980): J. Immunol., 125:2810-2817.
34. Wagner, H., Hardt, C., Heeg, K., Rollinghoff, M., and Pfizenmaier, K. (1980): Nature, 284:278-280.
35. Walford, R. (1974): Fed. Proc., 33:2020-2027.
36. Welte, K., Wang, C.Y., Mertelsmann, R., Venuta, S., Feldman, S.P., and Moore, M.A.S. (1982): J. Exp. Med., 156:454-464.
37. White, B.A., and Bancroft, F.C. (1982): J. Biol. Chem., 257:8569-8572.
38. Wiskocil, R., Weiss, A., Imboden, J., Kamin-Lewis, R., and Stobo, J. (1985): J. Immunol., 134:1599-1603.
39. Wu, W., Pahlavani, M.A., Cheung, H.T., and Richardson, A., Cell. Immunol., (submitted).
40. Yoshida, T. (1979): In: Biology of Lymphokines, edited by S. Cohen, E. Pick, and J.J. Oppenheim, pp. 259-290. Academic Press, New York.

ADVERSE DRUG INTERACTIONS IN THE ELDERLY

Timothy R. McNamara

St. Louis College of Pharmacy, and
Program on Aging, Jewish Hospital of St. Louis
St. Louis, Missouri 63178

A drug interaction can be defined as an unintended response that is directly attributable to the actions of two or more drugs causing either toxicity or therapeutic failure. Drugs have many different physiologic effects. These depend not only upon a drug's specific action at receptor sites, but also upon independent physiologic responses in patients. It is often difficult to determine when an observed response or lack thereof, is actually due to an interaction between drugs. In the elderly, this is further compounded by the unpredictability in the degree of physiologic changes that occur with age.

This chapter is intended as an introduction to: a) discuss a review of the theoretical considerations which put the elderly patient more at risk for drug interactions; b) examine some of the studies which report the incidence and factors related to adverse drug interactions in the elderly; and c) offer suggestions which will help to facilitate safe and effective drug utilization in this population.

THEORETICAL BASIS FOR ADVERSE DRUG INTERACTIONS

As can be seen in Table 1, there are numerous mechanisms for drug interactions. Detailed reviews of these mechanisms, complete with examples, are available elsewhere in the literature (1,17,18). Because the physiologic changes that occur in aging affect both the pharmacokinetics and pharmacodynamics of drugs in this population, this review will discuss the implications of these changes as potential causes for drug interactions.

Pharmacokinetic interactions are caused by changes in drug disposition, i.e., altered absorption, distribution, metabolism and elimination. For example, the interaction between phenylbutazone and warfarin can result in excessive anticoagulation and hemorrhage. This is because both drugs are highly protein bound and, therefore, are not widely distributed outside of the plasma. By displacing warfarin from protein binding sites, the amount of free (active) drug is increased resulting in a more active drug being available to elicit an effect. Conversely, the continuation of warfarin with phenobarbital can potentially cause a decreased anticoagulant effect, due to the ability of phenobarbital to stimulate the hepatic metabolism of warfarin.

Pharmacodynamic interactions occur when two or more drugs act at the same receptor site or affect the same physiologic systems. These effects can be additive when drugs have similar actions or opposite when their actions oppose each other. One example of an added pharmacodynamic interaction would be excessive central nervous system depression caused by drugs which possess this property such as anticholinergics, phenothiazines, benzodiazepines and ethanol. An opposite pharmacodynamic interaction is represented by the concomitant use of antihypertensive medications and over-the-counter decongestants which contain sympathomimetics such as pseudoephedrine. The sympathetic stimulations caused by nasal decongestants will often negate that of the antihypertensive, leading to increased dosage requirements and increasing the potential for toxicity.

TABLE 1. Mechanisms of drug interactions

1. Pharmacokinetic
   a. direct chemical or physical interactions
   b. interactions in gastrointestinal absorption
   c. interactions due to accelerated or inhibited metabolism
   d. interactions due to effects elicited by previously administered drugs

2. Pharmacodynamic
   a. interactions at the receptor site
   b. interactions due to previously administered drugs

The important physiologic changes associated with altered pharmacokinetics in the elderly are those related to altered drug distribution and elimination. A detailed review of pharmacokinetics and aging can be found elsewhere (8).

The elderly undergo changes in body composition which lead to a reduction in total body water and lean body mass, and an increase in the percentage of total body fat content (5). These changes can be expected to decrease the volume of distribution of water soluble drugs and to cause the opposite effect on those drugs which are fat soluble. These effects have been demonstrated in elderly humans where water soluble ethanol was found to have higher plasma concentrations without changes in the metabolic rate (28), while valium had an increased initial and total steady-state volume of distribution (12). Both of these changes are thought to at least partially account for an increased sensitivity to these two agents in the elderly.

Changes in the elimination of drugs with aging is most significant in relation to renal clearance. An average decline of 35 percent in glomerular filtration rate is known to occur between the ages of 20 and 90 years, and both glomerular and tubular function are affected (20). Reduced drug dosage requirements in association with age-related decreases in renal clearance have been observed for digoxin (7), cimetidine (24), and gentamicin (22).

Distribution and elimination changes in the elderly are further magnified when one considers the potential for drugs to interact with each other. For example, if a particular drug decreases glomerular filtration rate, its effects can be expected to be of greater significance in a person with already impaired renal function. When combined with other drugs which undergo renal elimination, excessive accumulation and toxicity might ensue. Digitalis is one agent which has previously been mentioned as having an age-related reduction in renal clearance. When used in combination with other drugs which cause an unpredictable decrease in renal function, such as the nonsteroidal anti-inflammatory agents, unexpected digitalis toxicity may occur.

The issue of pharmacodynamic changes in the elderly is less well-studied. Clinical trials have documented that the elderly are less responsive to the effects of isoproterenol and propranolol on heart rate (16,29), while being more sensitive to benzodiazepines (3,9,19) and potent analgesics (11). The additive effects of drugs with sedative properties is one of the most common interactions observed clinically in the elderly.

Another factor in the elderly which might be expected to alter pharmacodynamics is the development of impaired homeostatic mechanisms (27). This has been documented for impaired glucose tolerance (6) and for regulation of body temperature (8). Examples of adverse drug reactions and interactions which could occur in association with these homeostatic changes include excessive hypoglycemia involving oral hypoglycemic agents, and hypothermia due to neuroleptic drugs (phenothiazines and butyrophenones).

An intangible factor which makes both pharmacokinetic and pharmacodynamic changes even more unpredictable is the clinical manifestations which are exhibited in response to illnesses. Rowe (21) has defined four factors contributing to this as: a) variability in the underlying physiologic changes; b) the other diseases which an individual has accumulated over time; c) the varying degrees of severity of pathologic processes; and d) the individual's pattern of response to illness and interactions with the health professionals. Thus, it can be postulated that if these factors can affect the clinical manifestations of disease, that they might have an impact upon the individual responses patients have to medications. Taking this one step further, these factors also might be expected to contribute to the adverse responses which can occur as a result of drug therapy.

In summary, there are multiple factors which can, at least in theory, account for increased susceptibility to adverse drug reactions and interactions in the elderly. Because of the variability of these factors, health practitioners must develop an increased awareness that any unpredictable or unexpected response to medications might be due to an adverse drug reaction or interaction.

THE INCIDENCE AND CAUSATIVE FACTORS FOR DRUG INTERACTIONS IN THE ELDERLY

The elderly take more drugs (13,26) and experience more adverse reactions (9,14,23) than the young. This is to be expected in a population that suffers from more chronic diseases and is exposed to a larger number of prescribers. The actual incidence of adverse reactions varies from 8.7 percent (14) to 21.3 percent (10) for ages 70-79, to as high as 24 percent (23) for ages 80 years and older. Levy et al. (15) have shown that a decline in the average number of medications prescribed for patients is associated with a decrease in the average number of adverse reactions. In the group 60 years and older, the average number of drugs decreased from 7.8 to 6.9 per person, and the rate of adverse reactions from 24.3 percent to 7 percent.

Compared to the reports which document the incidence of adverse drug reactions in the elderly, there are few studies which document the incidence of adverse drug interactions. A Canadian study (2), utilizing a home care team to determine drug therapy through medical records and home interviews, reported 78 potential drug interactions involving 34 percent of 150 patients 65 years and older. Cooper et al. (4) identified potential drug interactions in 23.4 percent of 562 patients in a study of seven nursing homes. Stanazek and Franklin (25) reported that 23 percent of 3028 outpatients at a Veterans Administration facility were at risk of potential drug interactions. A total of 935 potential interactions were identified out of the 12,836 drugs prescribed. The population greater than 60 years old accounted for 35 percent of the potential interactions and 23 percent of the study population.

While these studies report that there is a high potential for drug interactions in the elderly population, none reported the incidence of clinically significant interactions, i.e., those interactions which lead to actual adverse clinical responses. They also failed to include interactions resulting in a lack of clinical response as potential interactions.

Other similarities in the studies occurred in the actual drug involved in the majority of interactions reported. These include digitalis (thiazide diuretics), antidiabetic agents (thiazides), antacids with phenothiazines and tetracycline, drugs with additive central nervous system depressant properties, digitalis (propranolol), and drugs with anticholinergic properties.

Even though the evidence presented suggests that the elderly are at a higher risk for potential drug interactions, there is a lack of evidence in well-designed studies which documents the actual incidence and severity of interactions. Until such studies can be carried out, health care providers must assume that the data that associate both increasing age and numbers of drugs with increased adverse reactions and potential interactions is valid. Thus, extra care must be taken when considering medication usage in the elderly.

CONCLUSIONS

The following recommendations should help to decrease the number of adverse drug interactions and reactions in the elderly.

1. Become familiar with the pharmacology of drugs, so that treatment regimens can be designed which take into account age and disease related changes in drug disposition.

2. Design a treatment plan with specific therapeutic endpoints and a time frame for desired therapeutic responses. Evaluate the necessity for the continuation of medications on a regular basis.

3. Prescribe the fewest drugs possible.

4. Obtain a thorough drug history which includes "over-the-counter" medications. If necessary, have the patient bring all of their drugs into the clinic, make a site visit, or obtain the history from a person responsible for overseeing the care of the patient.

5. Recommend to the patient that they use the same physician and pharmacy for their health care needs.

6. Provide the patient or caregiver with explicit directions for drug use.

7. Use drugs with distinct physical features (colors and shapes) when possible.

8. Avoid, when possible, using drugs with similar side effects or a high incidence of adverse reactions or interactions.

9. When an undesired or unexpected clinical event occurs, suspect that it may be drug related, and carefully review the patient's medications for potential interactions or adverse reactions.

Prescribers now have available to them information documenting age- and disease-related changes which can affect drug disposition. Also, evidence indicates that reductions in the numbers of medications patients receive is associated with a decrease in drug related morbid events. By approaching drug treatment in the elderly patient with the above-mentioned concepts in mind, safer and more effective drug therapy in the geriatric patient should be achieved.

REFERENCES

1. Aarons, L. (1981): Pharmacol. Ther., 14:321-344.
2. Blondeau, F., Fabia, J., Doyon, F., Demers, D., Brosseau, J., and Perrault, H. (1984): Union Med. Can., 113:666-670.
3. Castelden, C.M., George, C.F., Marcer, D., and Hallet, C. (1979): Br. Med. J., 1:10-12.
4. Cooper, J.W., Wellins, I., Fish, K.H., and Loomis, M.E. (1975): J. Am. Pharm. Assoc., 15:24-31.
5. Crooks, J., O'Malley, K., and Stevenson, I.H. (1976): Clin. Pharmacokinet., 1:169-180.
6. Davidson, M.B. (1979): Metabolism, 28:688-690.
7. Ewy, G.A., Kapadia, G.G., Yao, L., Lullian, M., and Marcus, F.I. (1974): Circulation, 39:30-42.
8. Fox, R.H., MacGibbon, R.D., Davies, L. (1973): Br. Med. J., 1:21-25.
9. Greenblatt, D.S., Allen, M.D., and Shader, R.I. (1977): Clin. Pharmacol. Ther., 21:355-361.
10. Hurwitz, N., and Wade, O.L. (1969): Br. Med. J., 1:539-540.
11. Kaiko, R.F. (1980): Clin. Pharmacol. Ther., 28:823-825.
12. Klotz, V., Avant, G.R., Hoyompa, H., Shenker, S., and Wilkinson, G.R. (1975): J. Clin. Invest., 55:347-359.
13. Levy, M., Ketter-Hemo, D., Nir, I., and Eliankim, M. (1977): Isr. J. Med. Sci., 13:1065-1069.
14. Levy, M., Kewitz, H., Altwein, W., Hillebrand, J., and Eliankim, M. (1980): Eur. J. Clin. Pharmacol., 17:25-31.
15. Levy, M., Lipsitz, M., and Eliankim, M. (1979): Am. J. Med. Sci., 277:49-56.
16. Londen, G.M., Safar, M.E., Weiss, Y.A., and Millier, P.L. (1976): J. Clin. Pharmacol., 16:174-182.
17. Morrelli, H.F., and Melmon, K.L. (1982): In: Clinical Pharmacology, edited by H. Melmon and K. Morelli, p. 982. McMillan, New York.
18. Pullman, C.C., and Stewart, R.B. (1985): In: Pharmacy Practice for the Geriatric Patient, edited by B. Ameer, J.L. Bootman, C. Brown, M.D. Higbee, W.F. McGhen and F.B. Palumbo, Chapter 12. Health Sciences Consortium, Inc., Carrboro, North Carolina.
19. Reidenberg, M.M., Levy, M., Warner, H., Coutinho, C.B., Schwartz, M.A., Yu, G., and Cherpico, I. (1978): Clin. Pharmacol. Ther., 23:371-375.
20. Rowe, J.W. (1976): J. Gerontol., 35:155-163.
21. Rowe, J.W. (1984): Psychosomatics, 25 (suppl.):6-11.

22. Sawchuck, R.J., Zaske, D.E., Cipolle, R.J., Wargin, W.A., and Strate, R.G. (1976): Clin. Pharmacol. Ther., 21:362-369.
23. Seidl, L.G., Thronton, G.F., Smith, J.W., and Cluff, L.E. (1966): Bull. Johns Hopkins Hosp., 119:299-315.
24. Shentag, J.J., Caller, G., Rose, J.Q., Cerra, F.B., DeGlopper, E., and Berhard, H. (1979): Lancet i:177-181.
25. Stanazek, W.F., and Franklin, C.E. (1978): Hosp. Pharmacol., 13:255-263.
26. Stewart, R.B., and Cluff, L.E. (1971): Johns Hopkins Med. J., 129:319-331.
27. Vestal, R.E. (1984): In: Drug Treatment in the Elderly, edited by R. Vestal, p. 35. Adis Health Sciences Press, Boston, Massachusetts.
28. Vestal, R.E., McGuire, E.A., Tobin J.D., Andres, R., Norris, A.A., and Mezey, G. (1977): Clin. Pharmacol. Ther., 31:343-354.
29. Vestal, R.E., Wood, A.J., and Shand, D.G. (1979): Clin. Pharmacol. Ther., 26:181-186.

VASCULAR ADRENERGIC RESPONSIVENESS IN AGING

Sue Piper Duckles

Department of Pharmacology, California College of Medicine, University of California, Irvine, California 92717

It is well-established that circulating plasma norepinephrine levels increase with age in humans (2,4,12,35,49). However, the interpretation of this finding is not clear-cut. Some authors interpret the increase in plasma norepinephrine as reflecting an increase in sympathetic activity with age, referring to the "hyperadrenergic state" of old age (39). In contrast, other authors assert that "the results of each of several different types of investigation are all compatible with the interpretation that the effectiveness of adrenergic stimulation declines with advancing age" (27).

In the case of cardiac function, there is abundant evidence suggesting that beta-adrenergic responsiveness declines with increasing age (23,26,28). Norepinephrine levels of the heart decline with age (20,37), and responses of isolated hearts to adrenergic agonists decrease with age (48).

ANIMAL STUDIES

Beta-adrenergic responsiveness of arterial smooth muscle also declines with age, although the greatest decline occurs before maturity (15,16,25). A continued decline in responsiveness of the aorta and pulmonary artery to beta-adrenergic stimulation has been shown as animals age beyond maturity (34), although other workers demonstrate a complete loss of beta-adrenergic relaxation of rat arteries by six months of age (10).

In contrast, beta-adrenergic relaxation of veins is not altered with age. Both rabbit and rat portal veins, as well as the rabbit renal vein, show a persistence of beta-adrenergic relaxation with age (14,15). As illustrated in Table 1, this is also true for the rat jugular vein (10). Sensitivity to isoproterenol as well as the propranolol dissociation constant, a measure of receptor affinity, does not change in jugular veins from rats 3 to 27 months of age. Thus, effects of age on beta-adrenergic mechanisms depend on the type of vessel studied: arteries show a rapid decline in beta-adrenergic responsiveness while beta-adrenergic responses remain strong in veins.

TABLE 1. Effect of age on sensitivity to isoproterenol and affinity for propranolol of the rat jugular vein[a]

Animal age	Isoproterenol (EC_{50})[b] $(\times 10^{-9} M)$	Propranolol (K_b)[c] $(\times 10^{-9} M)$
3	6.8 (3.6-12.9)	ND[d]
6	6.9 (4.5-10.7)	3.3 ± 0.8
12	6.5 (5.3- 7.9)	2.8 ± 0.5
20	10.0 (6.2-16.2)	3.4 ± 1.1
27	4.0 (1.7- 9.3	3.0 ± 0.8

[a]Data from Duckles and Hurlbert (10).
[b]Concentration to produce 50 percent of maximum response. Geometric mean and 95 percent confidence interval were determined by method of Fleming et al. (17).
[c]Propranolol dissociation constant determined by the method of Furchgott (18).
[d]ND = not determined.

Literature concerning the effect of age on alpha-adrenergic responsiveness of blood vessels is much less clear-cut. As reviewed by Fleisch (14), changes in responsiveness to alpha-adrenergic stimulation have been reported by some authors while others have found no alteration with age. However, few investigators have verified the specificity of alterations in alpha-adrenergic receptor responses by testing other less specific contractile agonists. Alterations in the magnitude of maximum contractile responses can reflect changes in vessel elasticity or smooth muscle structure, rather than specific changes in alpha-adrenergic responsiveness. Use of large conducting vessels, such as the aorta, makes this problem even more likely to occur (44).

Another difficulty with many studies of aging is the failure to include the full life span of the animal. Thus, many studies of "aging" are really studies of maturation, as senescent animals are not included. Additionally, many studies do not include enough age groups. The study of one "old" and one "young" group of animals can be misleading if the young animals are not fully mature or if the old group includes a greater proportion of diseased animals (7). Age-related changes should begin at maturity and show a continued decline into senescence.

Several authors have reported that norepinephrine content of blood vessels declines with age in human (33,45) as well as rat (13) vessels. However, a recent study suggests that this may not always be true. While norepinephrine content declined with age in the rat renal, femoral, and saphenous arteries, there was no age-related decline in norepinephrine content in the superior mesenteric artery (24).

One cannot assume from norepinephrine content alone that function of the adrenergic neuroeffector will change correspondingly. Compensatory adaptations may occur so that operation of the unit as a whole may be unchanged. Furthermore, norepinephrine content by itself may not be an adequate measure of functional adrenergic activity (11). Indeed, measurement of [^{3}H]norepinephrine accumulation, an alternative indicator of adrenergic nerve functional activity, indicates that adrenergic activity is well-maintained with advancing age. Neuronal [^{3}H]norepinephrine accumulation is unchanged with age in the femoral artery and renal artery and vein (9). In the femoral vein, neuronal [^{3}H]norepinephrine accumulation is higher at 6 and 27 months of age than at 12 and 20 months. Thus, function of the entire neuroeffector mechanism must be assessed in order to determine how aging affects its operation.

One way to assess the function of the adrenergic neuroeffector mechanism as a unit is to determine the sensitivity to transmural nerve stimulation in vitro. These determinations were made for the rat femoral artery and vein and rat renal artery and vein (9). Frequency response curves showed that, on the whole, sensitivity to adrenergic nerve stimulation does not alter with age. There was one exception to this: the rat femoral vein showed a significantly greater contractile response to stimulation at 4 Hz than femoral veins from older animals. However, this does not change the overall conclusion that adrenergic responsiveness does not decline with advancing age, as there was no progressive decline from 12 to 27 months of age, and as shown by animal weight, 6-month-old rats are not fully grown.

Analysis of maximum responses also indicated that adrenergic responsiveness was well-maintained through senescence (9) (Table 2). Thus, there was no age-related decline in the ability of these arteries and veins to contract when assessed either as maximum response to norepinephrine or as maximum response to the nonspecific stimulus, 150 mM KCl. Furthermore, if maximum responses to transmural nerve stimulation are analyzed as a percent of maximal norepinephrine responses, there were no age-related changes (9). These data suggest that the overall ability of the tissue to respond to adrenergic nerve stimulation is well-maintained with age.

TABLE 2. Maximum contractile responses in vitro for rat vessels as a function of age[a]

	Grams Developed Force			
	6 mos.	12 mos.	20 mos.	27 mos.
Femoral artery				
TNS[b]	0.73+0.09	0.81+0.10	0.98+0.11	0.86+0.09
NE	1.10+0.12	1.11+0.16	1.45+0.09	1.33+0.13
KCl	1.05+0.11	0.92+0.21	1.16+0.09	0.96+0.13
Femoral vein				
TNS	0.85+0.10	0.89+0.07	0.75+0.04	0.86+0.12
NE	0.82+0.05	1.00+0.09	0.83+0.03	0.96+0.10
KCl	0.55+0.07	0.67+0.08	0.50+0.04	0.59+0.07
Renal artery				
TNS	1.23+0.10	1.43+0.16	1.25+0.20	1.08+0.12
NE	1.35+0.14	1.59+0.16	1.45+0.25	1.36+0.12
KCl	0.84+0.07	1.03+0.11	0.97+0.19	0.82+0.10
Renal vein				
TNS	0.49+0.07	0.73+0.13	0.73+0.07	0.69+0.11
NE	0.49+0.08	0.68+0.08	0.68+0.06	0.64+0.08
KCl	0.28±0.03	0.47±0.07	0.42±0.04	0.41±0.07

[a]Data from Duckles et al. (9).
[b]TNS = Transmural nerve stimulation; NE = norepinephrine

Analysis of responses to exogenous norepinephrine suggest that this is due in part to maintenance of responses mediated by alpha-adrenergic receptors (9). Thus, analysis of concentration response curves to norepinephrine in the carotid and femoral arteries indicate that sensitivity to alpha-adrenergic stimulation does not change with age. The concentration of norepinephrine to produce 50 percent of a maximal response (EC_{50}) was constant in vessels from rats 6 to 27 months of age.

Analysis of sensory innervation of the vasculature reveals a different pattern of age-related changes. Levels of substance P in mesenteric arteries and veins show a rise with age (Table 3) (8). In the mesenteric artery, substance P levels rise at 22 months of age while in the vein, substance P levels were increased at 20 months of age and were 75 percent higher at 27 months of age than at 6 months.

While the presence of substance P-containing primary sensory afferent innervation of the vasculature has been clearly shown (19), the function of these nerves is not well understood. The most extensively explored function of vascular substance P-containing nerves is the response to antidromic stimulation of sensory afferents in the skin and eye, including vasodilation and plasma extravasation (29,30). Although substance P can increase blood flow and can relax vascular smooth muscle through an endothelium-dependent mechanism (3,38), the significance of an increase in substance P content with age is not clear. This could reflect an increased density of substance P nerves or, perhaps more likely, an increased substance P content of each nerve ending. Whether this might represent a build-up of substance P content due to decreased nerve activity or result in an actual increase in functional activity of the sensory system with age requires further study.

TABLE 3. Effect of age on substance P levels of rat mesenteric artery and vein[a]

	Substance P content (pmoles/g)			
	6 mos.	12 mos.	20 mos.	27 mos.
Mesenteric artery	4.8+1.0	3.5+0.3	5.1+0.4	9.1+0.6[b]
Mesenteric vein	8.3±1.8	7.3±0.8	10.9±0.6[c]	14.5±0.6[d]

[a]Data from Duckles (8).
[b]Different from 6, 12, and 20 months, $p < 0.0006$.
[c]Different from 12 months, $p < 0.02$.
[d]Different from 6 and 12 months, $p < 0.02$.

Thus, the following conclusions can be drawn about the effects of age on vascular reactivity in the rat model. First of all, the magnitude and sensitivity to beta-adrenergic relaxation shows a sharp decline in arteries, with much of this occurring before maturity. In contrast, in veins, there is no decline with age in sensitivity to beta-adrenergic relaxation. As far as sensitivity to alpha-adrenergic stimulation, this is well-maintained into advancing age, with the magnitude of maximal contractile response also maintained.

Norepinephrine content declines with age in some vessels, but not invariably. Assessment of [^{3}H]norepinephrine accumulation, an alternative measure of adrenergic nerve function, shows no decline with age. The lack of decline in function of the adrenergic neuroeffector junction is further supported by measurements of contractile responses to adrenergic nerve stimulation in vitro. In both arteries and veins studied, there are no age-related declines in either sensitivity to adrenergic nerve stimulation or maximum response. Thus, an overall conclusion is that function of the adrenergic neuroeffector mechanism is well-maintained with age in the rat. An important caveat to this conclusion is that these studies have focused on a very discrete aspect of the entire system for blood pressure control. Alterations at other sites, such as baroreceptor sensing, central control, or ganglionic transmission, could result in profound changes in overall cardiovascular function even though function of the adrenergic nerve ending vascular smooth muscle complex is well-maintained.

HUMAN STUDIES

An important question to be asked about studies using the rat model is how applicable are these conclusions to man? Given the limitations of techniques available to assess cardiovascular function in humans, there is relatively little on which to base an answer. However, available information does suggest that the rat is a good model for man in this regard.

Sensitivity to norepinephrine of arteries isolated from humans ranging from 30 to 83 years of age does not change with age (40,42). When expressed as a percent of maximum responses to KCl, maximum responses to norepinephrine do not decline with age (40,42). However, in males, but not in females, maximum responses to KCl and norepinephrine, expressed as grams force, do decline with age, reflecting structural alterations with increasing age. These findings suggest that alpha-adrenergic mechanisms are well-maintained with age in the human vasculature.

The stability of vascular adrenergic responses with age is also supported by the findings of two clinical studies in humans (31,41). Since the evidence of postural hypotension is higher among older individuals (47), the cause of postural hypotension was investigated. While there was evidence of a decline in autonomic function in the elderly, this was no greater in patients with postural hypotension. Thus, a change in vascular structure, most likely due to arteriosclerosis, was the probable cause of postural hypotension in these patients. It was felt most likely that alterations in sympathetic activity were central in origin, rather than peripheral (31,41).

At the present time, it is difficult to say what the significance of these age-related changes in vascular adrenergic responsiveness might be. In most cases, one can only speculate. For example, it is intriguing to find that in veins, beta-adrenergic relaxation is well-maintained from maturity to old age in contrast to what has been shown for arteries. Although little is known about the function of beta-adrenergic receptors in a large vein such as the jugular, we would hypothesize that this vessel may serve as a model for venous beta-adrenoceptors in general. Specific venous segments containing a predominance of beta-adrenoceptors have been demonstrated in the rabbit (36) and the rat (6). It has been hypothesized that these venous segments participate in redistribution of blood flow to facilitate thermoregulation (46). In that case, maintenance of function during aging would be an important benefit to the organism.

HOMEOSTASIS AND VASCULAR RESPONSE

It is remarkable that, both in humans and animals, many elements of vascular adrenergic reactivity are so well-preserved in advancing age. However, it has been shown that a key change that does occur with advancing age is a loss of adaptability. For example, both central hemodynamic parameters and blood flow to several different regions are not different when conscious 24-month-old rats are compared to 12-month-old animals (43). However, when animals are anesthetized with pentobarbital, senescent rats showed a much greater susceptibility to the stresses of anesthesia and surgery. Anesthesia produced significantly greater reductions in blood flow to several organs in 24-month-old rats than in 12-month-old animals.

There are a number of other examples of studies showing a reduced ability of older animals to adapt to stressful situations. After catecholamine depletion with reserpine, many regions of the central nervous system show an increased number of beta-adrenergic receptors. However, in aged rats, this response to chemical denervation is obtunded (22). It has also been shown that increased numbers of beta-adrenergic receptors develop in the pineal gland after exposure to light. This alteration in tissue responsiveness does not occur in aged rats (21).

Studies have also been done to assess the cardiovascular response of aged rats to acute immobilization stress (5). The blood pressure of adult rats increased significantly during a brief immobilization but this did not occur in aged rats. The cardiovascular response to stress of old rats was delayed or diminished although there was an exaggerated exhaustion phase which continued irreversibly to death within 24 hours in all of the aged rats studied. Several authors have also shown that older rats are not as capable of adjusting to acute cold stress as are young rats (1,32).

From these studies, it is possible to predict that although the adrenergic responsiveness of the vasculature may not be changed in the resting state, the addition of stress to the animal will reveal a reduced activity of adaptive mechanisms. Further studies must be done to explore the separate factors involved in maintaining cardiovascular homeostasis in order to document the specific deficits in aged animals that result in reduced cardiovascular adaptability.

ACKNOWLEDGMENTS

Supported by a grant from the National Institutes of Health, AGO 6080 and by an Established Investigatorship from the American Heart Association.

REFERENCES

1. Balmagiya, T., and Rozovski, S.J. (1983): Exp. Gerontol., 18:199-210.

2. Barnes, R.F., Raskind, M., Gumbrecht, G., and Halter, J.B. (1982): J. Clin. Endocrinol. Metab., 54:64-69.
3. Bury, R.W., and Mashford, M.L. (1977): Eur. J. Pharmacol., 45:335-340.
4. Christensen, N.J. (1983): Acta Med. Scand. (Suppl.), 676:52-63.
5. Chuieh, C.C., Nespor, S.M., and Rapoport, S.I. (1980): Neurobiol. Aging., 1:157-163.
6. Cohen, M.L., and Wiley, K.S. (1978): J. Pharmacol. Exp. Ther., 205:400-409.
7. Duckles, S.P. (1983): Neurobiol. Aging, 4:151-156.
8. Duckles, S.P. (1985): Neurobiol. Aging, 6:237-239.
9. Duckles, S.P., Carter, B.J., and Williams, C.L. (1985): Circ. Res., 56:109-116.
10. Duckles, S.P., and Hurlbert, J.S. (1986): J. Pharmacol. Exp. Ther., 236:71-74.
11. Duckles, S.P., and Rapoport, R. (1979): J. Pharmacol. Exp. Ther., 211:219-224.
12. Embree, L.J., Roubein, I.F., Jackson, D.W., and Ordway, F. (1981): Exp. Aging Res., 7:215-224.
13. Esler, M., Skews, H., Leonard, P., Jackman, G., Bobik, A., and Korner, P. (1981): Clin. Sci., 60:217-219.
14. Fleisch, J.H. (1980): Pharmacol. Ther., 8:477-487.
15. Fleisch, J.H., and Hooker, C.S. (1976): Circ. Res., 38:243-249.
16. Fleisch, J.H., Maling, H.M., and Brodie, B.B. (1970): Circ. Res., 26:151-162.
17. Fleming, W.W., Westfall, D.P., De la Lande, I.S., and Jellette, L.B. (1972): J. Pharmacol. Exp. Ther., 181:339-345.
18. Furchgott, R.E. (1972): In: Catecholamines: The Classification of Adrenoceptors, edited by H. Blaschko and E. Muscholl, pp. 283-335. Springer-Verlag, New York.
19. Furness, J.B., Papka, R.E., Della, N.G., Costa, M., and Eskay, R.L. (1982): Neuroscience, 7:447-459.
20. Gey, K.F., Burkard, W.P., and Pletscher, A. (1965): Gerontologia, 11:1-11.
21. Greenberg, L.H., and Weiss, B. (1978): Science, 201:61-63.
22. Greenberg, L.H., and Weiss, B. (1979): J. Pharmacol. Exp. Ther., 211:309-316.
23. Guarnieri, T., Filburn, C.R., Zitnik, G., Roth, G.S., and Lakatta, E.G. (1980): Am. J. Physiol., 239:H501-H508.
24. Handa, R.K., and Duckles, S.P. (1985): Fed. Proc., 44:1109.
25. Hayashi, S., and Toda, N. (1978): Br. J. Pharmacol., 64:229-237.
26. Kreider, M.S., Goldberg, P.B., and Roberts, J. (1984): J. Pharmacol. Exp. Ther., 231:367-372.
27. Lakatta, E.G. (1980): Fed. Proc., 39:3173-3177.
28. Lakatta, E.G., Gerstenblith, G., Angell, C.S., Shock, N.W., and Weisfeldt, M.L. (1975): Circ. Res., 36:262-269.
29. Lembeck, F. (1983): Trends Neurosci., 6:106-107.

30. Lembeck, F., and Holzer, P. (1979): N-S. Arch. Pharmacol., 310:175-183.
31. MacLennan, W.J., Hall, M.R.P., and Timothy, J.I. (1980): Age Ageing, 9:25-32.
32. McCarty, R. (1985): J. Autonom. Nerv. Syst., 12:15-22.
33. Neubauer, B., and Christensen, N.J. (1978): Gerontology, 24:299-303.
34. O'Donnell, S.R., and Wanstall, J.C. (1984): J. Pharmacol. Exp. Ther., 228:733-738.
35. Palmer, G.J., Ziegler, M.G., and Lake, C.R. (1978): J. Gerontol., 33:482-487.
36. Pegram, B.L., Bevan, R.D., and Bevan, J.A. (1976): Circ. Res., 39:854-860.
37. Rappoport, E.B., Young, J.B., and Landsberg, L. (1981): J. Gerontol., 36:152-157.
38. Regoli, D., D'Orleans-Juste, P., Escher, E., and Mizrahi, J. (1984): Eur. J. Pharmacol., 97:161-170.
39. Rowe, J.W., and Troen, B.R. (1980): Endocrinol. Rev., 1:167-179.
40. Scott, P.J.W., and Reid, J.L. (1982): Br. J. Clin. Pharmacol., 13:237-239.
41. Smith, S.A., and Fasler, J.J. (1983): Age and Ageing, 12:206-210.
42. Stevens, M.J., Lipe, S., and Moulds, R.F.W. (1982): Br. J. Clin. Pharmacol., 14:750-752.
43. Tuma, R.F., Irion, G.L., Vasthare, U.S., and Heinel, L.A. (1985): Am. J. Physiol., 249:H485-H491.
44. Tuttle, R.S. (1966): J. Gerontol., 21:510-516.
45. Waterson, J.G., Frewin, D.B., and Soltys, J.S. (1974): Blood Vessels, 11:79-85.
46. Winquist, R.J., and Bevan, J.A. (1980): Science, 207:1001-1002.
47. Wollner, L., and Spalding, J.M.K. (1978): In: Textbook of Geriatric Medicine and Gerontology: The Autonomic Nervous System, edited by J.C. Brocklehurst, pp. 245-267. Churchill Livingstone, New York.
48. Yin, F.C.P., Spurgeon, H.A., Greene, H.L., Lakatta, E.G., and Weisfeldt, M.L. (1979): Mech. Ageing Dev., 10:17-25.
49. Ziegler, M.G., Lake, C.R., and Kopin, I.J. (1976): Nature, 261:333-335.

LIVER DRUG METABOLISM DURING AGING: RODENT VS PRIMATE MODELS

Douglas L. Schmucker

Cell Biology and Aging Section and the Intestinal Immunology Research Center, Veterans Administration Medical Center, and Department of Anatomy and the Liver Center, UCSF School of Medicine, San Francisco, California 94143

The fact that aging results in a marked decline in overall drug disposition has been fairly well—established (see 31, 49 for reviews). However, the mechanism(s) primarily responsible for this reduced adaptive capacity remain unresolved. Arguments have been made for and against age-related changes in drug absorption, drug distribution, drug metabolism and drug excretion as major contributors to reduced disposition in the elderly (see 36, 37 for reviews). Although there is a paucity of evidence demonstrating altered drug absorption during aging, considerable support has been generated for the other three parameters.

Many drugs and xenobiotics are metabolized in one of several organs including the liver, kidney, small intestine, and lungs, prior to their elimination or clearance. Since the liver is the primary site of drug metabolism and many drugs undergo mandatory biotransformation by the liver microsomal mixed-function oxidase system (MFOS), this pathway has been subjected to considerable scrutiny as a function of aging. Unfortunately, the clinical data on this issue are somewhat controversial and difficult to interpret due to inherent methodological problems in many of the studies. Although there are conflicting reports, a number of studies have demonstrated significantly prolonged plasma half-lives for a variety of drugs metabolized by the hepatic MFOS in geriatrics vs young adults (Table 1; see 9, 32 for reviews). However, there are major problems with much of these data including (a) marked interindividual variation, e.g., as much as a sixfold range in the clearance rate of antipyrine; and (b) the lack of correlation between such parameters as reduced liver blood flow, liver volume, drug clearance and subject age (see 48 for a review). Furthermore, there have been no definitive studies on in vitro liver drug metabolism in humans. The general consensus is that the evidence for an age-related decline in liver Phase I MFOS function(s) in humans is circumstantial (see 37 for a review).

TABLE 1. Age-dependent alterations in the plasma half-lives of various drugs in humans

Drug	Age range[a] (years)	Plasma half-life (hours)	Reference
Phenobarbital	30 - 70	20 - 107	17
Antipyrine	26 - 78	12 - 17	28
Diazepam	20 - 70	20 - 80	22
Practolol	27 - 80	7 - 8.5	8
Digoxin	27 - 77	51 - 73	10

[a]Maximum ages examined

RODENT MODELS

Practically all of the data on in vitro drug metabolism as a function of aging has been obtained in highly inbred male rodent models. Kato et al. (20,21) are generally credited as being the first to demonstrate a negative correlation between chronological age and liver MFOS function(s). Subsequent studies from a number of different laboratories demonstrated age-dependent declines in: a) the in vivo and in vitro hepatic metabolism of various drugs; b) the noninduced activities of MFOS enzymes; and c) the inducibility of MFOS components by drugs in rodents (3,5,6,12,26,46). However, even in the rodent models there have been conflicting data with regard to in vitro liver MFOS activities (Table 2). Some of these apparent discrepancies may be attributable to differences in the sex, strain, or maintenance of the experimental animals. Regardless, two schools of thought emerged, one which suggested that aging

TABLE 2. Age-dependent alterations in the rat liver microsomal mixed-function oxidase system

Parameter measured	Age range[a] (months)	Alteration	Reference
Noninduced MFOS activities	1 - 27	Decline	39
Noninduced MFOS activities	3 - 25	Decline	34
Induced MFOS activities	3 - 30	No Change	5,6
Induced MFOS activities	2 - 24	No Change	19
Induced MFOS activities	7 - 31	Decline	26
Induced MFOS activities	1 - 27	Decline	34

[a]Maximum ages examined

caused a significant and irreversible decline in liver drug metabolism and another which espoused the concept that aging only minimally affected the hepatic MFOS and this effect was transient (Fig. 1). The central theme of this concept was that old animals exhibited a "lag" period between the administration of the MFOS-inducing agent and the initiation of MFOS enzyme/heme protein synthesis (1). Ultimately, the MFOS parameters, e.g., NADPH cytochrome $\underline{c}$ (P450) reductase, in the old subjects would be induced to the levels achieved in the young animals. Other investigators have been unable to detect such lag periods under similar experimental conditions, and their data tend to support the former hypothesis (4,41).

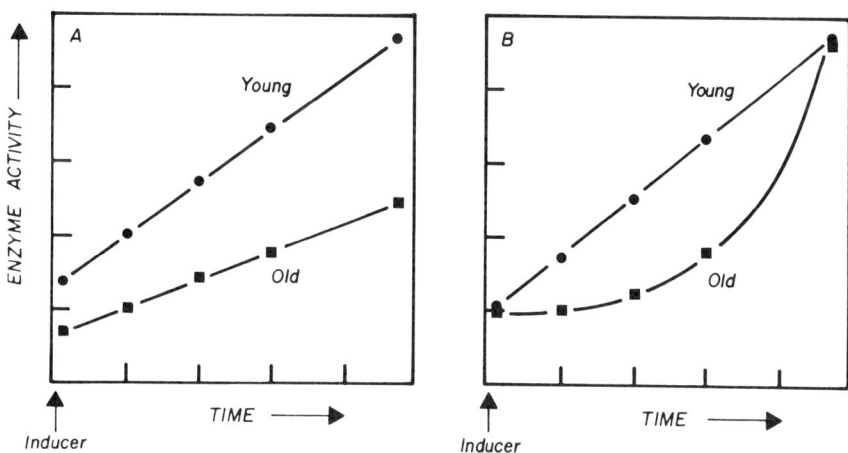

FIG. 1. Graphic representation of two major concepts of the effects of aging on liver microsomal drug metabolism in rodent models. The left panel (A) is based on the observations of Kato et al. (20,21) who reported that several MFOS parameters exhibited marked declines in both basal values and drug-induced activities. The horizontal axis illustrates the duration of MFOS induction with a drug, e.g., phenobarbital, and the vertical axis represents the activities of MFOS enzymes or heme proteins. In this model, even maximally induced MFOS values in senescent rats did not approach the levels achieved in drug-induced young animals. This model (B) is based on the observations of Adelman et al. (1) and maintains that the noninduced levels of MFOS activities in young and old rats are similar. Although there is a lag in the induction of MFOS activities which is age-dependent, the values attained in the maximally induced senescent animals are similar to those measured in similarly treated young adult rats.

AGE CHANGES IN LIVER MFOS COMPONENTS

Several important liver MFOS components in male Fischer 344 rats exhibit significant age-related decline (Fig. 2; 40,41). The specific activity of NADPH cytochrome $\underline{c}$ (P450) reductase, the concentration of the cytochromes P450 and the rate of ethylmorphine N-demethylation were reduced between two and fourfold in senescent rats in comparison to young or mature animals. Phenobarbital elicited marked increases in several MFOS parameters in young, mature, and senescent male rats, although the age-related differences between the basal values remained or were enhanced even after six days of drug treatment (Fig. 3; 41). Interestingly, the magnitude of most of the drug-induced increases was similar, e.g., four to fivefold for the cytochromes P450, regardless of animal age.

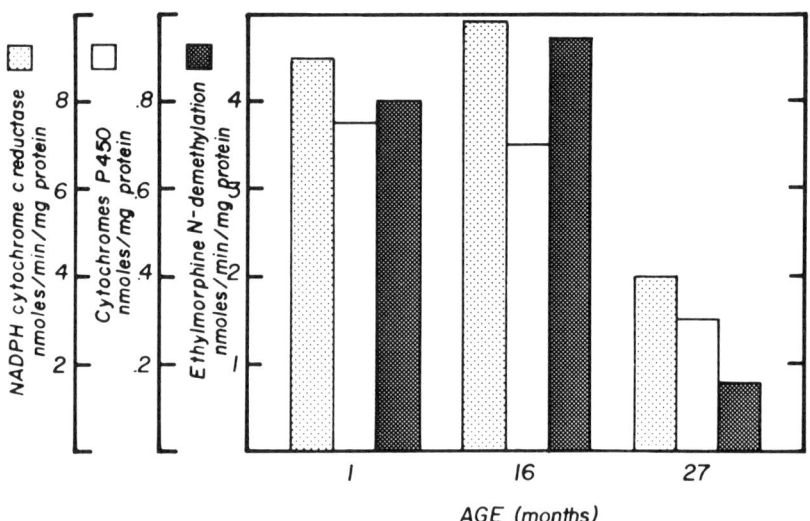

FIG. 2. Effect of aging on several rat liver MFOS parameters. Significant declines occur in the specific activity of NADPH cytochrome $\underline{c}$ (P450) reductase, the concentration of the cytochromes P450, and in the rate of ethylmorphine N-demethylation measured in vitro in isolated microsomes.

Collectively, the studies cited above suggest an age-dependent decline in the functional capacity of the liver microsomal MFOS, although the direct evidence is based largely on in vitro data from rodents and does not eliminate extrahepatic influences, e.g., shifts in steroid hormone levels. Furthermore, the cellular, subcellular, and molecular mechanism(s) responsible for this decline remain to be elucidated. Altered rates of hepatic drug metabolism may reflect qualitative or quantitative changes in critical MFOS enzymes or heme proteins which culminate in reduced catalytic efficiency (see 11, 35 for reviews). Alternative suggestions include the possibility that age-related alterations in the MFOS are due to perturbations in other MFOS components, e.g., the microsomal membrane (33).

The decline in liver drug metabolism measured in old rats may be due, in part, to a concomitant loss of the smooth surfaced endoplasmic reticulum membrane (SER), the primary site of the MFOS (Fig. 4). In fact, quantitative electron microscopic analysis revealed a 40-50 percent decline in the concentration of this hepatocellular membrane in male Fischer rats as a function of age (Fig. 5; 38). Interestingly, Pieri et al. (29) reported an age-related increase in this parameter

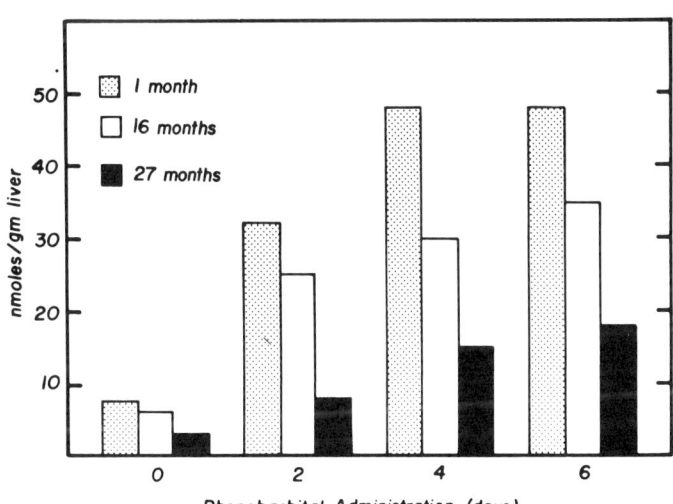

FIG. 3. Effect of aging on the inducibility of rat liver microsomal cytochromes P450. Male Fischer 344 rats at ages of 1, 16, and 27 months were subjected to phenobarbital administration (50 mg/kg/day) for up to 6 days and several important MFOS functions were measured in vitro. The age-dependent differences in the noninduced levels of the cytochromes P450 were maintained and, in fact, enhanced during phenobarbital treatment. At no time during the induction period did the concentration of the cytochromes P450 in either the mature or senescent rat livers approach the levels measured in the young adult animals.

in female Wistar rats. A subsequent study by Meihuizen and Blansjaar (27) also reported an increase of approximately 30 percent in the relative volume of SER in the livers of rats between 3 and 35 months of age. These conflicting data may be reconciled by the consideration of several facts: a) Pieri et al. did not employ preferred tissue preparative methods for stereological analysis; b) both Pieri et al. and Meihuizen and Blansjaar used female rats of different strains, whereas Schmucker and Wang (40) employed male Fischer animals; and c) Meihuizen and Blansjaar estimated the relative volume rather than the surface-to-volume ratio of SER--the former stereological parameter being of questionable value when applied to measurements of membrane sheets rather than particulate organelles. Lastly, the age-dependent decline in the amount of SER as measured by stereology correlates well with the yield of microsomal protein obtained from the livers of similarly aged rats (Fig. 5; 41).

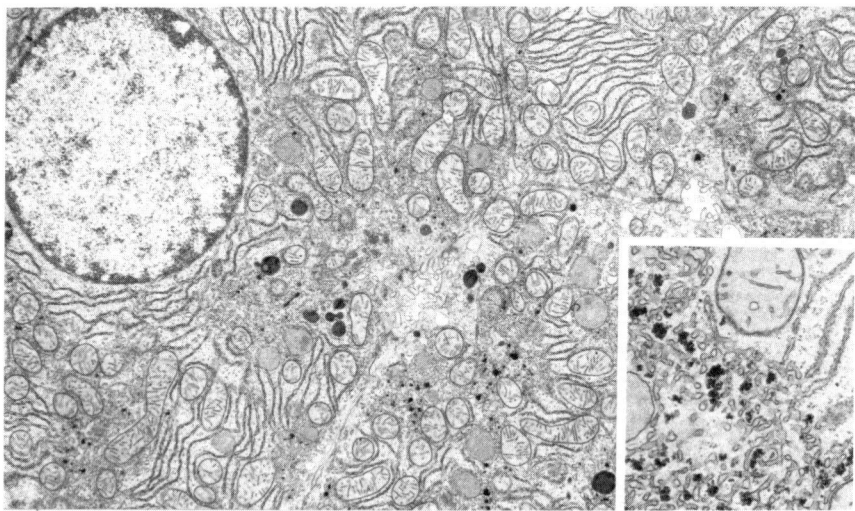

FIG. 4. Electron micrograph of typical hepatocytes from a young adult rat. The fine structural appearance of liver tissue from young and senescent animals was qualitatively similar except that the cells from old animals contained considerably more dense bodies (lysosomes, residual bodies). INSET: High magnification of SER in hepatocyte from the same animal. M, mitochondria; ly, lysosome; SER, smooth surfaced endoplasmic reticulum; RER, rough endoplasmic reticulum.

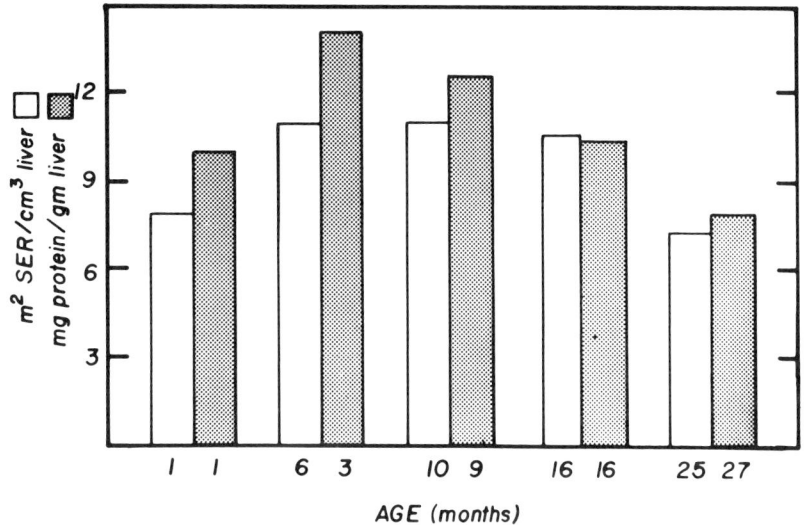

FIG. 5. <u>Age-dependent shifts in the hepatocellular concentrations of smooth SER and microsomal protein.</u> There is good correlation between these two parameters during aging in the Fischer rat. Each bar represents the mean value for at least five animals.

AGE CHANGES IN CATALYTIC EFFICIENCY OF MFOS ENZYMES

There is considerable evidence for an age-dependent accumulation of "altered" enzymes which exhibit diminished catalytic efficiency, e.g., rat liver aldolase and superoxide dismutase (see 11, 35 for reviews). A similar phenomenon may occur with MFOS enzymes and, therefore, may contribute to reduced liver drug metabolism. Although rat liver microsomal NADPH cytochrome $\underline{c}$ (P450) reductase undergoes a significant age-related decline in specific activity, the kinetic profile of the membrane-bound enzyme remains essentially unchanged during aging (Table 3; 43).

However, the enzyme from old rats was more sensitive to product inhibition with NADP than microsomal reductase from younger animals. A recent analysis of solubilized rat liver microsomal NADPH cytochrome $\underline{c}$ (P450) reductase demonstrated several specific age-related alterations in the quality of this important rate-limiting MFOS enzyme (42). The specific activity of the solubilized enzyme isolated from young adult animals and purified to homogeneity was twofold higher than that of similar preparations from other age groups (Fig. 6). Furthermore, there was: a) no change in the molecular weight; b) a shift to a more heat stable form; and c) no differences in cross-reactivity with antibody against "young" reductase. More importantly, the specific activity of the immunoprecipitable

TABLE 3. Effect of aging on the kinetic profile of rat liver microsomal NADPH cytochrome c (P450) reductase

	Animal ages (months)		
	3	16	27
K_m NADPH (μM)	6.9	6	6.5
V_{max} (x 10^{-2})	5	2.7	2.4
K_m cytochrome c (μM)	4	2.9	2.2
V_{max} (x 10^{-2})	3.2	3	2.4
K_i NADP (μM)	59	-	15

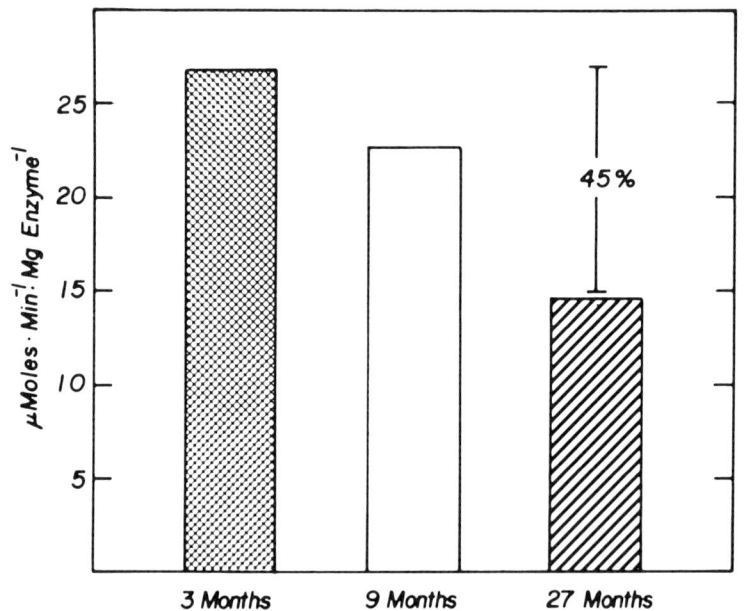

FIG. 6. Effect of aging on the specific activity of solubilized rat liver microsomal NADPH cytochrome c (P450) reductase. The enzyme was purified to homogeneity as determined by polyacrylamide gel electrophoresis and the activity was measured using cytochrome c as the terminal electron acceptor. Each bar represents the mean value for several pooled samples of purified enzyme.

TABLE 4. Effect of aging on the specific activity of immunoprecipitable rat liver microsomal NADPH cytochrome c (P450) reductase

	Animal ages (months)		
	3	9	27
Immunoprecipitation radius (mm)[a]	2	2	3.2
Enzyme protein per well (μgm)	.038	.045	.069
Enzyme activity (μmole/min)	0.1	0.1	0.1

[a]The radial immunodiffusion plate contained goat anti-rat NADPH cytochrome c (P450) reductase.

enzyme exhibited a significant age-dependent decline as measured by radial immunodiffusion and immunotitration (Table 4; 42).

The yield of purified enzyme from young adult rats represented approximately 50-60 percent of the total reductase complement. Subsequent calculations based on measurements of total enzyme activity and recovered enzyme protein suggested that the microsomes of old rats contained twice the enzyme content as those of younger animals (Table 5). When these values were corrected to reflect the relative yields of microsomal protein, there was essentially no difference in the amount of reductase per gram of liver tissue between young and old rats. Furthermore, the larger livers in mature and senescent animals contained considerably more enzyme in comparison to those of younger rats. In essence, the old rats contained more reductase in their livers, but at least half of the enzyme was "altered" or catalytically inefficient. These data support the possibility that the age-related decline in MFOS capacity results from changes intrinsic to the hepatocytes and, in particular, to MFOS constituents.

TABLE 5. Effect of aging on the hepatic content of microsomal NADPH cytochrome c (P450) reductase in rats

	Animal ages (months)		
	3	9	27
Enzyme yield (μgm/mg microsomal protein)	2	.8	.2
% Enzyme recovery	21	7	1-2
Estimated enzyme content (μgm/mg microsomal protein)	9.5	11.8	16.7
Corrected enzyme content (μgm/gm liver)	135	148	137
Corrected total enzyme content (μgm/liver)	797	1214	1370

MEMBRANE LIPIDS AND MFOS ACTIVITY

The demonstration of "altered" MFOS enzymes does not exclude alternative changes which may ultimately impair the efficiency of hepatic drug metabolism. Although aging appears to have little effect on the protein/polypeptide composition of the hepatic microsomes, several investigators have reported age-related changes in the lipid domain of this membrane system (13,15,53). Certain phospholipids influence the efficacy of MFOS enzymes, e.g., phosphatidylcholine is required for optional NADPH cytochrome P450 reductase activity. Therefore, shifts in the distribution profile of the major membrane phospholipids may impact on the metabolic capacity of the MFOS. In addition, an increase in the phosphatidylethanolamine/phosphatidylcholine ratio seems to have an inhibitory effect on microsomal reductase. Recent data from our laboratory demonstrated a slight decline in the phospholipid content of hepatic microsomes from senescent Fischer rats (Table 6; 44). An age-related increase in the cholesterol content of these same membranes contributed to concomitant increases in the cholesterol/phospholipid ratio and in the solidity of the lipid domain (Fig. 7).

TABLE 6. Effect of aging on the phospholipid composition of rat liver microsomes

	Animal age (months)		
	3	16	25-27
Phosphatidylcholine (μgm/mg microsomal protein)	10 ± 1.7	11.9 ± 3.1	9.1 ± 3.5
Phosphatidylinositol (μgm/mg microsomal protein)	1.9 ± 0.8	1.9 ± 0.7	1.4 ± 0.5
Phosphatidylethanolamine and phosphatidylserine (μgm/mg microsomal protein)	3.6 ± 1.0	5.2 ± 1.4	3.0 ± 0.8

The fatty acid composition of hepatic microsomes also exhibits changes as a function of aging. Grinna (13) reported an age-related increase in the most unsaturated species of fatty acid (C 22:6; decosahexaenoic) in rats. More recently, Hawcroft et al. (15) demonstrated marked declines in the relative proportions of oleic (C 18:1) and linoleic acids (C 18:2) in the microsomes of old mice vs those of younger animals, and this observation has been confirmed in our laboratory (44). Shifts in the concentrations of the more saturated fatty acid species, which constitute approximately 80 percent of the total pool, may influence the physical properties of the membranes, e.g., fluidity. However, the physiological impact of such changes remains unresolved. van Bezooijen (50) has presented much of the data concerning the effects of aging on the lipid composition of liver

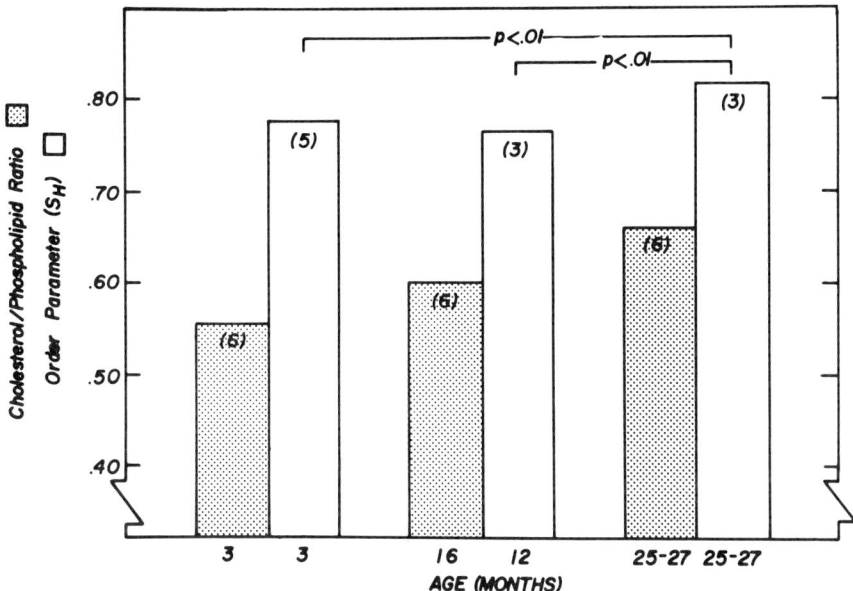

FIG. 7. <u>Effect of aging on the cholesterol/phospholipid ratio and the fluidity of the lipid domain of rat liver microsomal membranes.</u> The cholesterol/phospholipid ratio, an important index of membrane fluidity, undergoes a substantial increase during aging. This shift is accompanied by an increase in the order parameter (S_H), a measure of rigidity, of the membrane such that the microsomes of old rats are significantly more rigid than those prepared from either young, adult, or mature animals. ( ) denotes the number of animals per group.

microsomes in rodent models in tabular form. The well-documented, age-dependent decline in hepatic microsomal MFOS function(s) may result from a number of factors, including (a) a loss of SER membrane and/or MFOS constituents; (b) alterations in the quality of MFOS enzymes or heme proteins which consequently reduce their catalytic efficiency; (c) changes in the lipid milieu of MFOS; or (d) any combination of the above (Fig. 8).

In summary, recent data on hepatic drug metabolism have established that the specific activities and/or amounts of several important MFOS components undergo significant declines during aging, at least in rodents. In these models, there is now evidence to support the contention that changes intrinsic to the hepatocyte contribute to the decline in liver drug metabolism.

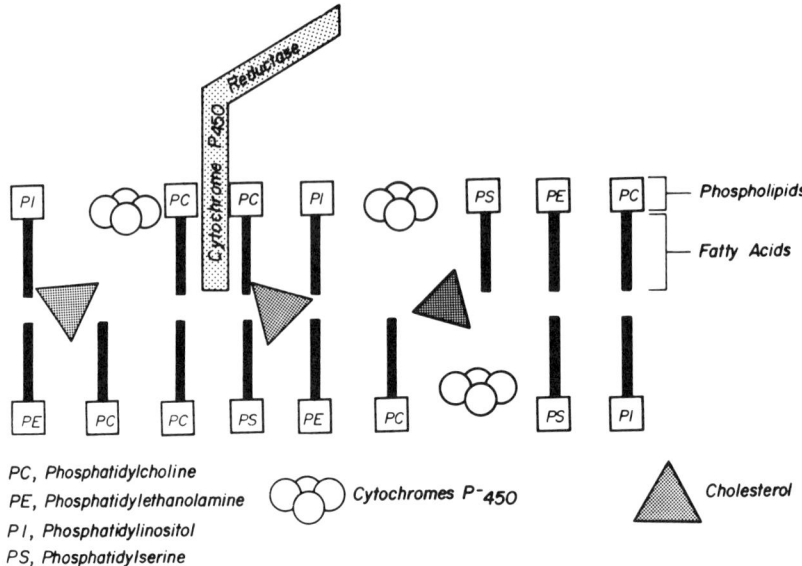

FIG. 8. Diagram of hepatic microsomal MFOS consisting of membrane lipid domain, NADPH cytochrome P450 reductase, and clusters of the cytochromes P450. Possible age-related alterations in these components include: a) the loss of important heme proteins, e.g., the cytochromes P450; b) reduced catalytic efficiency of NADPH cytochrome P450 reductase; c) reduced phospholipid/cholesterol ratio which may affect the efficiency of constituent enzymes, e.g., NADPH cytochrome P450 reductase; d) reduced fluidity of the lipid domain and subsequent impairment of the lateral mobility of enzymes and heme proteins. In addition, an age-related decline in cellular protective mechanisms against free radical attack, e.g., reduced levels of glutathione and lower activities of glutathion-s-transferases and superoxide dismutase, may permit higher rates of peroxidation of membrane lipids by superoxide radicals generated by MFOS itself.

Reidenberg (30) stated that "...the elderly appear to metabolize drugs at one-half to two-thirds the rate of young adults...". However, this generalization seems premature in view of: a) the paucity definitive supporting evidence; and b) the reported extreme variation in MFOS functional parameters within the geriatric population. A recent review by van Bezooijen (50) brings together much of these data on rodent models and places them in a reasonably proper perspective. The author emphasized: a) the potential impact of individual variation on human pharmacokinetic parameters; b) the relative absence of this factor in populations of highly inbred rodents, such as those usually employed in drug studies; and c) the obvious consequences of extrapolating data obtained in rodent models to humans. Similar cautions have been expressed regarding the relative merits of a longitudinal vs a cross-sectional approach to clinical pharmacological studies (52). With respect to this, Baird (2) recently suggested that the well-documented, age-related decline in rodent liver MFOS capacity may not be a universal feature of aging. The only available in vitro data on human liver microsomal MFOS function(s) suggest that the cytochromes P450 content is not reduced in elderly subjects (18). However, there are certain methodological problems inherent in this study which render the data difficult to interpret.

The influence of sex on the hepatic metabolism of drugs has received considerable attention during the past few years. The fact that sex differences influence liver drug metabolism has been documented in rodents and to some small extent in humans (see 14 for a review). Since the age-related decline in hepatic MFOS function is not as apparent in females, fluctuations in the serum levels of sex steroids have been implicated as a causative factor in males. Castration of male rats leads to a "feminization" of liver drug metabolism, as does the chronic administration of estrogens. The general consensus is that testosterone stimulates and estrogens slightly inhibit the hepatic MFOS. While reduced testosterone levels may influence liver drug metabolism in old male rats, e.g., shifts in the cytochromes P450 subpopulations, there is no direct evidence for androgenic control of the liver MFOS in humans. The only studies to date reported: a) a correlation between the plasma half-life for antipyrine, patient age, and serum testosterone levels in a population of male geriatrics (16); and b) the absence of any significant sex differences in a wide spectrum of in vitro liver MFOS functions in tissues from kidney donors (23). Even the data obtained in rodent models is conflicting. Rikans and Notley (34) were unable to enhance several liver MFOS parameters in senescent male rats by the administration of methyltestosterone. Evidence to the contrary has been reported by Bitar and Weiner (7) wherein testosterone treatment of castrated old rats restored the hepatic cytochromes P450 levels to those measured in intact young adult animals. These conflicting reports emphasize the paucity of data in this particular arena and the need for additional studies.

NONHUMAN PRIMATE MFOS ACTIVITY

The difficulties inherent in obtaining sufficient viable human liver tissue for adequate analyses of in vitro MFOS function(s) during aging has prompted two recent studies in nonhuman primates. Sutter et al. (47) measured several liver MFOS indices in female pigtailed macaques (M. nemestrina)

TABLE 7. Effect of aging on liver MFOS parameters in female Macaque nemestrina[a]

Animal ages (years)	Cytochromes P450 (nmols/mg protein)	Cytochrome P450 reductase (nmols/min/mg protein
2 - 5.5	2.14 ± .12	196 ± 16
10 - 12	1.90 ± .21	172 ± 19
16 - 21	2.05 ± .14	163 ± 12

[a]Values represent the mean ± SE for groups of 8 animals

ranging in age from 2 to 21 years. These investigators reported no significant age-related changes in the content of the cytochromes P450 or in the specific activity of NADPH cytochrome c (P450) reductase (Table 7). In addition, the in vitro metabolism of aryl hydrocarbons remained unchanged during aging.

In a very similar study using male and female rhesus monkeys (Macaque mulatta) between the ages of 1 and 25 years, Maloney et al. (24) observed results essentially identical to those of Sutter et al. (47). Although the cytochromes P450 content was unaffected by either aging or sex, the specific activity of microsomal NADPH cytochrome c (P450) reductase exhibited a substantial increase rather than a decline between the ages of 10 and 20 years (Figs. 9 and 10). However, the degree of individual variation was considerable and seemed to increase with age--an observation similar to that of James et al. (18) in humans.

In very preliminary studies in our laboratory, solubilized and purified hepatic microsomal NADPH cytochrome c (P450) reductase from male and female rhesus monkeys does not appear to undergo any marked changes in molecular weight or in its kinetic profile. On the other hand, the activity of the solubilized enzyme exhibits a concerted decline (approximately 50 percent) during aging--a phenomenon similar to that observed for the male rat liver enzyme (42). Concomitantly, the heat inactivation profile of the soluble reductase shifts to a more heat labile form suggesting the presence of an "altered" enzyme (see 11, 35 for reviews). Interestingly, this shift is opposite to that observed with the solubilized reductase from the livers of male Fischer 344 rats (42). Although there appear to be several indices of age-related changes intrinsic to monkey liver microsomal NADPH cytochrome c (P450) reductase, the preliminary nature of these observations precludes any more definitive statements.

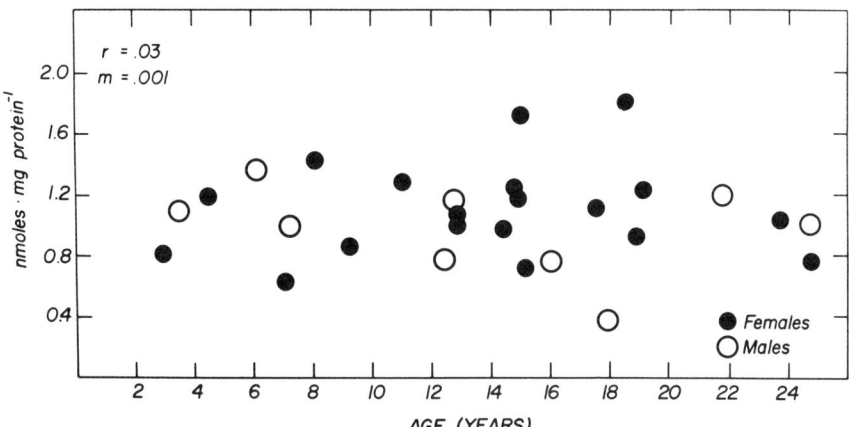

FIG. 9. Effect of aging on the concentration of cytochromes P450 in the hepatic microsomes of male and female rhesus monkeys. Both males and females exhibited similar patterns devoid of significant age-dependent shifts in heme protein levels although there was considerable variability in the values within narrow age ranges.

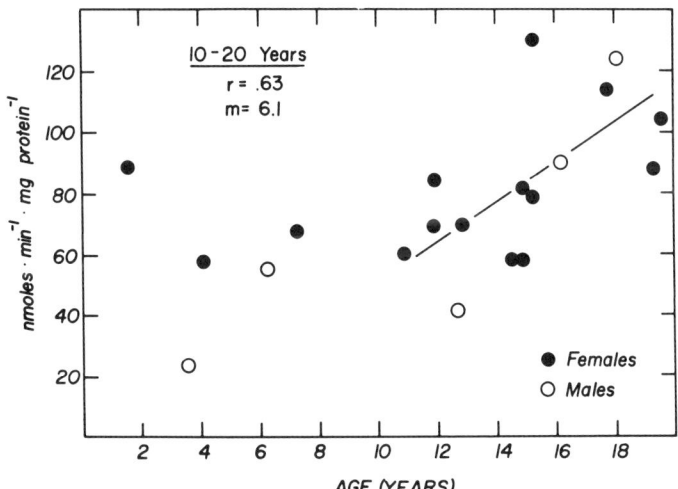

FIG. 10. Effect of aging on the specific activity of hepatic microsomal NADPH cytochrome c (P450) reductase from male and female rhesus monkeys. Enzyme activity exhibited a distinct increase during the latter half of the age span examined although the individual variation was considerable.

A number of investigators have suggested that the composition and/or fluidity of the microsomal lipid domain may influence the metabolic capacity of the hepatic MFOS (25,45,51). In view of the age-related shifts in these parameters in the rat liver MFOS, subsequent studies focused on similar indices in the monkey liver system. Neither the total phospholipid nor the cholesterol concentrations of the microsomes exhibited any marked age- or sex-related changes in the rhesus monkey (Fig. 11). There were no shifts in the relative distributions of the major classes of phospholipids. However, Sutter et al. (47) reported substantial age-related increases in microsomal phospholipid and cholesterol contents, 25 percent and 30 percent, respectively, in the pigtailed macaque. Therefore, the cholesterol/phospholipid ratio in these membranes remained virtually unchanged as a function of age. On the other hand, our data from the rhesus monkey model indicate a significant decline in this ratio during adulthood (approximately 25 percent), followed by a substantial increase during senescence (approximately 20 percent). Due to the lack of sufficient samples, no effort was made to determine the fatty acid composition or the saturation index of these membranes. Thus, the impact of any age- or sex-related shifts

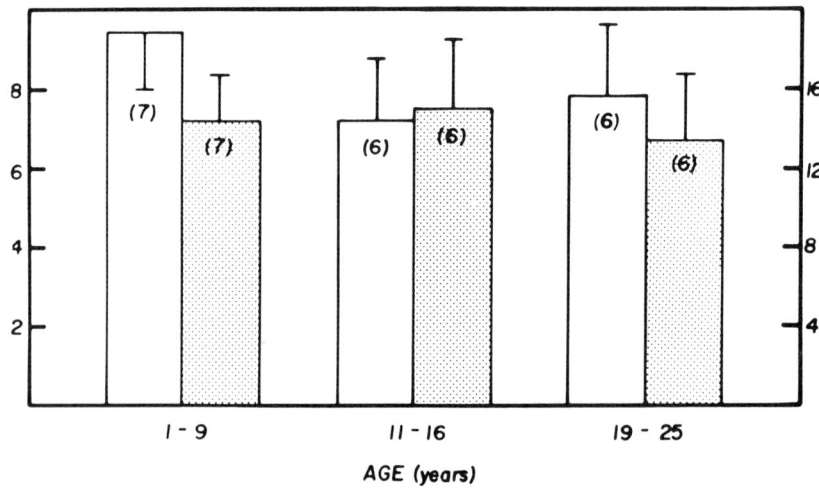

FIG. 11. <u>Effect of aging on the phospholipid and cholesterol contents of male and female rhesus monkey liver microsomes.</u> Although the shifts in the concentrations of these constituents are minor, they are reflected in rather marked changes in the cholesterol/phospholipid ratio. ( ) denotes the number of animals per age group; each bar reflects the mean values + the S.D. Cholesterol (unshaded) μgm/mg protein; phospholipid (shaded) μgm/Pi/mg protein.

in this parameter on membrane fluidity, and subsequently MFOS function(s), remain speculative. Still, the fluidity of the lipid domain of these membranes undergoes age-related shifts which correlate well with the changes in the cholesterol/phospholipid ratio (Table 8). The microsomes of young adult and senescent animals are considerably more rigid than those of mature monkeys ($p < .05$). Interestingly, the microsomes of senescent rats and monkeys are more rigid than the membranes of mature animals of both species (44). However, the correlation between decreased membrane fluidity and reduced hepatic MFOS function(s), which is apparent in the rat, is absent in the rhesus monkey model.

TABLE 8. Effect of aging on the cholesterol/phospholipid ratio and fluidity of monkey liver microsomes

Animal ages (years)	Cholesterol/ Phospholipid	Order Parameter (S_H)
1 - 9	.68 + .15	.735 + .05
10 - 16	.49 + .10	.650 + .06
19 - 25	.62 ± .22	.726 ± .02

CONCLUSION

The results expressed in this chapter demonstrate the problems inherent in extrapolating data on in vitro liver drug metabolism derived in inbred rodents to primates or humans. Furthermore, these data demonstrate quite clearly that individual variation must be considered a significant factor in any analysis of outbred populations. This observation demands particular attention inasmuch as most of the experimental data on the subject of age-dependent alterations in in vitro liver drug metabolism have been derived from highly inbred male rodents, such as the Fischer 344 rat. In this regard, the absence of any apparent sex-related differences in hepatic MFOS function(s) or in the physiochemical properties of the microsomes suggest that those reported in several rodent models may be species specific. In view of the above, perhaps emphasis should be directed toward the increased use of more appropriate animal models for aging studies, e.g., outbred rodent and primates of both sexes.

REFERENCES

1. Adelman, R. (1975): Fed. Proc., 34:179-182.
2. Baird, M. (1983): Exp. Gerontol., 18:47-53.
3. Baird, M., Samis, H., and Massie, H. (1971): Nature, 233:565-567.
4. Birnbaum, L. (1980): Exp. Gerontol., 15:259-267.

5. Birnbaum, L., and Baird, M. (1978): Exp. Gerontol., 13:299-303.
6. Birnbaum, L., and Baird, M. (1978): Exp. Gerontol., 13:469-477.
7. Bitar, M., and Weiner, M. (1983): Mech. Ageing Dev., 23:285-296.
8. Castledon, C., Kaye, C., and Parsons, R. (1975): Br. J. Clin. Pharmacol., 2:303-306.
9. Crooks, J., O'Malley, K., and Stevenson, I. (1976): Clin. Pharmacokinet., 1:280-296.
10. Ewy, G., Kapadia, G., Yao, L., Lullin, M., and Marcus, F. (1969): Circulation, 39:449-453.
11. Gershon, D. (1979): Mech. Ageing Dev., 9:189-196.
12. Gold, G., and Widnell, C. (1974): Biochim. Biophys. Acta, 334:75-85.
13. Grinna, L. (1977): Mech. Ageing Dev., 6:197-205.
14. Gustafsson, J., Mode, A., Norstedt, G., and Skett, P. (1983): Ann. Rev. Physiol., 45:51-60.
15. Hawcroft, D., Jones, T., and Martin, P. (1982): Arch. Gerontol. Geriatr., 1:55-74.
16. Higuchi, T., Nakamura, T., and Uchino, H. (1980): J. Natl. Cancer Inst., 65:887-900.
17. Houghton, G., Richens, A., and Leighton, M. (1975): Br. J. Clin. Pharmacol., 2:251-256.
18. James, O., Rawlins, M., and Woodhouse, K. (1982): In: Liver and Ageing--1982, edited by K. Kitani, pp. 395-408. Elsevier, North Holland, Amsterdam.
19. Kao, J., and P. Hudson. (1980): Biochem. Pharmacol., 29:1191-1194.
20. Kato, R., and Takanaka, A. (1968): J. Biochem. (Tokyo), 63:406-408.
21. Kato, R., Vasanelli, P., Frontino, G., and Chiesara, E. (1964): Biochem. Pharmacol., 13:1037-1051.
22. Klotz, U. (1975): J. Clin. Invest., 55:347-359.
23. Kremers, P., Beaune, P., Crestell, T., DeGraeve, J., Columelli, S., Leroux, J-P., and Gielen, J. (1981): Eur. J. Biochem., 118:599-606.
24. Maloney, A., Schmucker, D., Vessey, D., and Wang, R. (1985): Hepatology, in press.
25. McElhaney, R., editor (1982): Current Topics in Membranes and Transport. Academic Press, New York.
26. McMartin, D., O'Connor, J., Fasco, M., and Kaminsky, L. (1980): Toxicol. Appl. Pharmacol., 54:411-419.
27. Meihuizen, S., and Blansjaar, N. (1980): Mech. Ageing Dev., 13:111-118.
28. O'Malley, E., Crook, J., Duke, E., and Stevenson, I. (1971): Br. Med. J., 3:607-609.
29. Pieri, C., Nagy, I.Z., Guili, C., and Mazzufferi, G. (1975): Exp. Gerontol., 10:291-304.
30. Reidenberg, M. (1980): Bull. NY Acad. Med., 56:287-294.

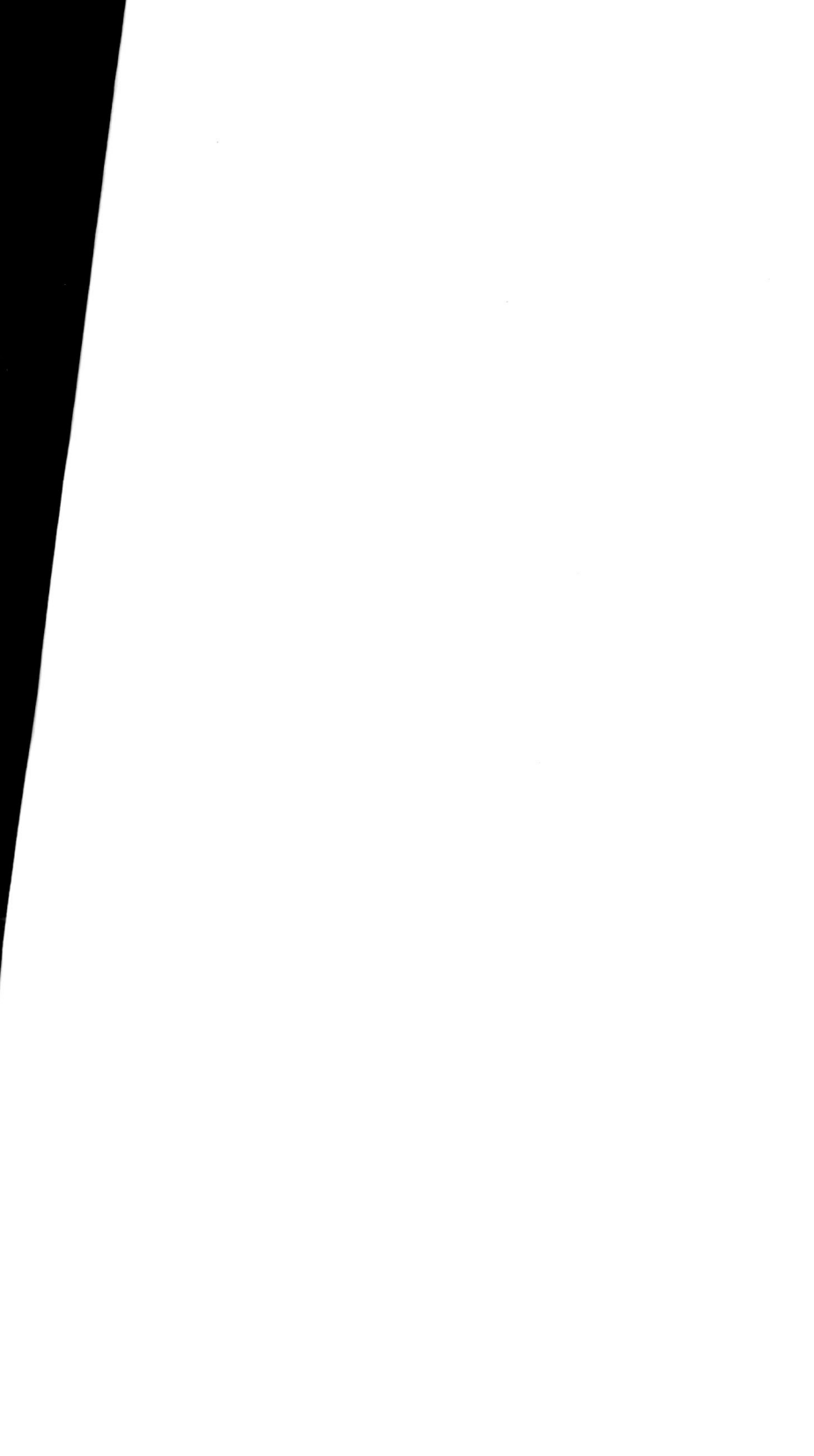

31. Richey, D. (1975): In: The Physi(of Human Aging, edited by R. Gc pp. 59-93. Academic Press, New
32. Richey, D., and Bender, A. (1977): Toxicol., 17:49-65.
33. Rikans, L., and Notley, B. (1982): Ther., 202:574-578.
34. Rikans, L., and Notley, B. (1984): M 25:335-341.
35. Rothstein, M. (1979): Mech. Ageing De
36. Schmucker, D. (1979): Pharmacol. Rev.,
37. Schmucker, D. (1985): Pharmacol. Rev.,
38. Schmucker, D., Mooney, J., and Jones, A Biol., 78:319-337.
39. Schmucker, D., and Wang, R. (1980): Exp. 15:321-329.
40. Schmucker, D., and Wang, R. (1980): Proc. Med., 165:178-197.
41. Schmucker, D., and Wang, R. (1981): Mech. 15:189-202.
42. Schmucker, D., and Wang, R. (1983): Mech. A(21:137-156.
43. Schmucker, D., and Wang, R. (1983): Exp. Gerc 18:313-321.
44. Schmucker, D., Wang, R., Vessey, D., James, J. Maloney, A. (1984): Mech. Ageing Dev., 27:20
45. Sonderman, H. (1978): Biochim. Biophys. Acta,
46. Stohs, S., Al-Turk, W., and Hassing, J. (1980): 3:88-92.
47. Sutter, M., Wood, W., Williamson, L., Strong, R. K., and Richardson, A. (1985): Biochem. Pharmac 34:2983-2987.
48. Triggs, E., and Nation, R. (1975): J. Pharmacokine Biopharm., 3:387-418.
49. Trounce, J. (1975): Br. J. Clin. Pharmacol., 2:289-
50. van Bezooijen, K. (1984): Mech. Ageing Dev., 25:1-2.
51. Vessey, D., and Zakim, D. (1982): In: Horizons in Biochemistry and Biophysics, edited by E. Quaglier P. Palmieri and T. Singer, pp. 139-162. Addison-Wes Press, Reading, Massachusetts.
52. Vestal, R. (1982): J. Am. Geriatr. Soc., 30:191-200.
53. Vlasuk, G., and Walz, F. (1982): Arch. Biochem. Biophys 214:248-259.

AGE-RELATED CHANGES IN THE ADENYLATE CYCLASE SYSTEM-- PHARMACOLOGICAL AND HORMONAL IMPLICATIONS

H. James Armbrecht and Philip J. Scarpace*

Geriatric Research, Education, and Clinical Center,
Veterans Administration Medical Center,
Departments of Internal Medicine and Biochemistry,
St. Louis University School of Medicine,
St. Louis, Missouri 63125;
*Geriatric Research, Education, and Clinical Center,
Veterans Administration Medical Center,
Sepulveda, California 91343, and Department of Medicine,
UCLA School of Medicine, Los Angeles, California 90024

One of the characteristics of aging is decreased responsiveness of some target tissues to hormones and drugs (9). This includes some of the hormones and drugs whose action is mediated by cAMP. For example, older adults have a lower heart rate response to isoproterenol when compared to mature adults, and the dose of isoproterenol required to increase the resting heart rate by 25 bpm increases with age (22). The capacity of parathyroid hormone to stimulate the renal production of 1,25-dihydroxyvitamin D, the biologically active metabolite of vitamin D, also declines with age in humans (21). Age-related changes in the action of isoproterenol (3) and parathyroid hormone (7) are seen in the rat as well.

The process by which hormones and drugs stimulate cAMP production and exert their physiological effects is complex. The steps involved include binding of the agonist to plasma membrane receptors, activation of adenylate cyclase to produce cAMP, activation of cAMP-dependent protein kinases, and phosphorylation of specific proteins. Age-related changes at any of these steps could result in age-related changes in hormone and drug action.

In the past few years, it has become clear that there are significant age-related changes in several parts of the pathway, including membrane receptor binding and activation of adenylate cyclase. Therefore, this chapter will summarize some of these age-related changes in systems that have been especially well-studied. In particular, the question of whether there is a common age-related defect in all systems or whether the defect varies from system to system will be addressed. The possible relevance of these age-related changes in adenylate cyclase to the overall decline in hormone and drug action will also be evaluated.

COMPONENTS OF THE ADENYLATE CYCLASE SYSTEM

The hormone receptor-coupled adenylate cyclase complex consists of at least three components (Fig. 1) (11,12,20). Located on the outer membrane surface is the receptor component containing a specific site for the binding of drugs and hormones. A hormone receptor (R) may either stimulate (R_s) or inhibit (R_i) enzyme activity. The second component of the system consists of the guanine nucleotide-binding regulatory proteins (N_s and N_i). These proteins are involved in both the stimulation (N_s) and inhibition (N_i) of adenylate cyclase activity. The third component of enzyme complex is the catalytic unit (C) which is the site of conversion of adenosine triphosphate (ATP) to adenosine 3', 5'-cyclic phosphate (cAMP).

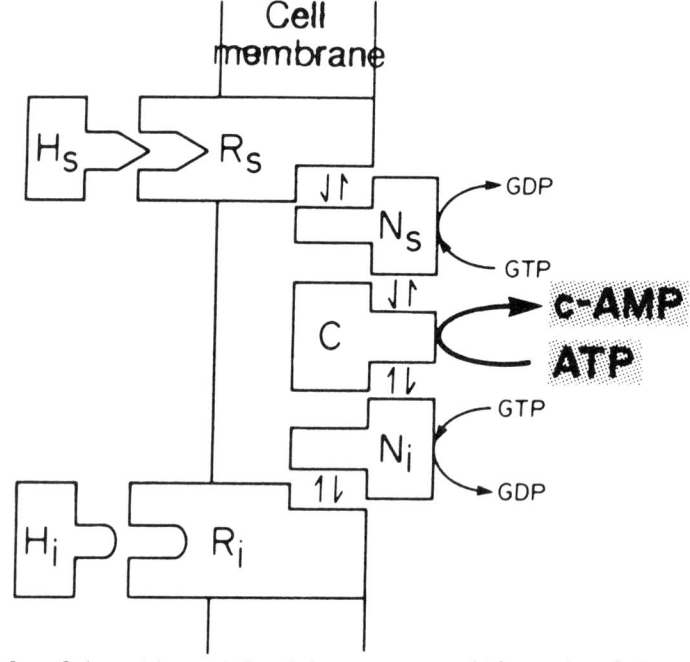

FIG. 1. Schematic model of hormone-sensitive adenylate cyclase system. ATP, adenosine triphosphate; C, catalytic unit; cAMP, adenosine 3',5'-cyclic phosphate; GDP, guanosine 5'-diphosphate; GTP, guanosine 5'-triphosphate; H, hormone; i, inhibitory; N, guanine nucleotide regulatory component; R, receptor; s, stimulatory. Figure taken from reference 20.

The sequence of events which leads to hormone activation of adenylate cyclase activity is complex and yet to be fully elucidated. The binding of hormone (H) to a stimulatory receptor (R_s) promotes the binding of R_s to N_s, thus forming the agonist high affinity complex (HRN_s). In the presence of guanosine 5'-triphosphate (GTP), the HRN_s complex is converted to N_s-GTP and HR. The active enzyme complex GTP-N_sC is then formed, and this complex converts ATP to cAMP. The lifetime of this active complex is regulated by a GTPase activity which converts GTP-N_sC to GDP-N_s and C (11,12,20). In an analogous fashion, an inhibitory hormone (H_i) may act through an inhibitory receptor (R_i) and the inhibitory guanine nucleotide regulatory component (N_i) to inhibit the conversion of ATP to cAMP by the catalytic unit.

THE ADRENERGIC SYSTEM--HUMAN LYMPHOCYTES AND PLATELETS

The beta-adrenergic stimulated adenylate cyclase activity of human lymphocytes has been well-studied as a function of age (2,13,14). The response of human lymphocytes to isoproterenol declines with age (Table 1) (2,13). This decreased responsiveness is not due to changes in total receptor number per cell (4). However, there is a decrease in agonist affinity. In particular, there is a decrease in the number of high affinity receptors in old subjects as compared to young subjects (8).

TABLE 1. Effect of age on adenylate cyclase activity of human lymphocytes, rat heart, and rat lung membranes[a]

Agonist	Age	Adenylate cyclase activity (pmol cAMP/mg protein/min)		
		Human lymphocytes	Rat heart	Rat lung
Isoproterenol (100 μM)	Young	96 ± 11	57 ± 9	60 ± 11
	Old	42 ± 10	45 ± 3	27 ± 5
NaF (10 mM)	Young	312 ± 59	47 ± 3	208 ± 2
	Old	62 ± 20	37 ± 6	115 ± 8
Forskolin (33 μM)	Young	352 ± 75	58 ± 7	124 ± 13
	Old	99 ± 22	39 ± 6	70 ± 6

[a]Data from human lymphocytes (2), rat heart (14,15), and rat lung (16) represent the mean ± SE of 5, 18, and 8 determinations, respectively. $P < 0.01$ (lymphocytes), $P < 0.05$ (heart) and $P < 0.005$ (lung) for differences with age. (One way analysis of variance)

In addition to changes in receptor affinity, age-related changes in lymphocyte N-protein function and/or catalytic unit function may contribute to decreased adenylate cyclase responsiveness. The decrease in sodium fluoride (NaF) and forskolin-stimulated adenylate cyclase activity with age (Table 1) supports this concept. NaF stimulates adenylate cyclase activity by acting on the N-protein, while forskolin stimulates by acting at the catalytic unit.

N-protein function was assessed in an <u>in vitro</u> complementation assay using the genetically N-protein-deficient membranes of cyc⁻ S49 mouse lymphoma cells (2,14). In this assay, N-protein was lubrol-extracted from the test tissue and combined with the mutant cells which were deficient in N-protein. In this manner, the added N-protein complemented the other components in the mutant cell line, leading to a complete enzyme complex. The extent of adenylate cyclase stimulation in the complemented mutant cells was a measurement of extracted N-protein. Human lymphocyte N-protein, as assessed by this assay, was not different between young and elderly subjects (2).

Catalytic unit activity was assessed by forskolin-stimulated adenylate cyclase activity. Forskolin is a cardioactive diterpere isolated from the roots of <u>Coleus Forskolii</u> and has been described as a direct activator of the catalytic unit (19). Forskolin-stimulated enzyme activity was reduced with age (Table 1), suggesting that the decrease in catalytic unit activity accounts for the observed decrease in enzyme activity. These age-related changes in the beta-adrenergic responsiveness of human lymphocytes are summarized in Table 4.

Since there are age-related changes in the beta-adrenergic adenylate cyclase system, it was of interest to determine if there were compensatory changes in the alpha-adrenergic system. Using human platelets, the alpha-adrenergic system has been studied as a function of age. Alpha-adrenergic compounds modulate adenylate cyclase activity through the alpha-2-adrenergic receptor and N_i (Fig. 1). Alpha-2-adrenergic receptors were assessed in human platelet membranes using the alpha-2-antagonist, yohimbine (1). There were no differences in the number or affinity of alpha-2-adrenergic receptors of young and elderly subjects. In addition, there were no age-related differences in the inhibition of adenylate cyclase activity by epinephrine in the presence of beta-adrenergic blockage. Thus, the age-related changes in the beta-adrenergic adenylate cyclase complex are neither augmented nor compensated for by changes in the alpha-2-adrenergic system.

THE ADRENERGIC SYSTEM--RAT HEART AND LUNG

Isoproterenol-stimulated adenylate cyclase activity of rat heart (15) and lung (16) membranes also decreases with age (Table 1). As with the human lymphocyte receptor, there were no age-related differences in the number of beta-adrenergic receptors of either lung or heart membranes (3,16). However, there were less receptors in the high-affinity state in older animals compared to younger animals for both heart (17) and lung (16). As shown in Table 2 for the lung membranes, the affinity for isoproterenol declines with age when binding to both high and low affinity sites is measured. However, low affinity binding does not change with age. Low affinity binding was determined by measuring the dissociation constant in the presence of guanyl-5-ylimidodiphosphate (GppNHp), which converts the HRN complex to the low affinity HR complex (see Fig. 1). Since low affinity binding does not change with age, the age-related decrease must be in the high affinity sites. The data suggest an inability of older animals to form the high-affinity binding complex.

Experiments were performed to determine if there were changes in the N-protein and the catalytic unit of rat heart and lung membranes. In each tissue, there was a decrease in NaF-stimulated enzyme activity with age (Table 1). This suggests that there are post-receptor changes in the adenylate cyclase system in this tissue. N-protein function was assessed in the in vitro complementation assay previously described. N-protein extracted from rat myocardial membranes demonstrated a progressive decrease in activity with age (Fig. 2) (14). Catalytic unit activity, as assessed by forskolin stimulation, also decreased with age in heart and lung (Table 1). This suggests that there are changes in the catalytic unit of both tissues with age. These changes in the beta-adrenergic responsiveness of rat heart and lung with age are summarized in Table 4.

TABLE 2. Apparent dissociation constants of beta-adrenergic receptor in lung membranes for isoproterenol[a]

	Dissociation constant (10^{-7} M)	
Age	High and Low Affinity Sites	Low Affinity Sites
3 mo	2.1 ± 0.3	4.2 ± 0.8
12 mo	2.6 ± 0.2	4.0 ± 0.5
24 mo	3.9 ± 0.4	4.4 ± 0.7

[a]Isoproterenol dissociation constants were determined from isoproterenol competition with [^{3}H]dihydroalprenolol (16). Data represent the mean ± SE of six animals. $P < 0.005$ (high and low affinity sites) for differences with age (t-test).

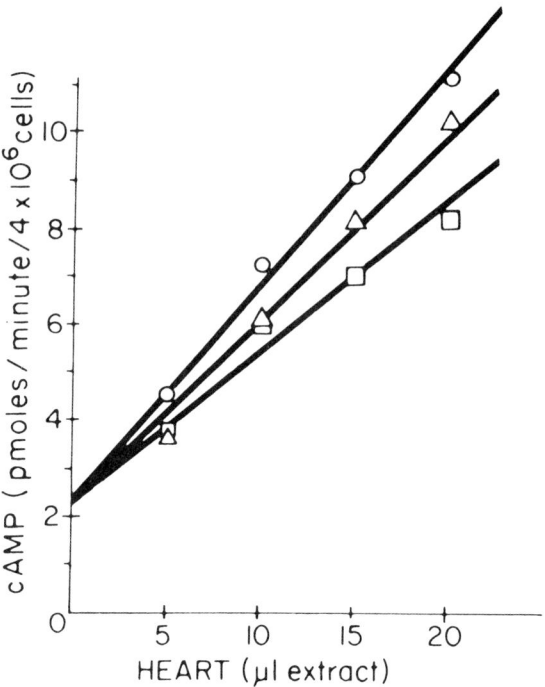

FIG. 2. N-protein activity in myocardial membranes from 3-(o), 12-(△), and 24-(□)-month-old rats. NaF-stimulated adenylate cyclase activity was determined following the addition of 0-20 µl of myocardial membrane extract to cyc⁻ membranes derived from 4×10^6 cells. Data represent duplicate determinations from a single animal in each age group. Figure taken from reference 14.

THE PARATHYROID HORMONE AND CALCITONIN SYSTEM--RAT KIDNEY

Parathyroid hormone-stimulated adenylate cyclase activity of rat renal cortical membranes declines with age (Table 3). In this tissue, the age-related changes appear to reside in the receptor. There were no age-related changes in the stimulation of adenylate cyclase by Gpp(NH)p or forskolin (Table 3). Gpp(NH)p is a nonhydrolyzable analog of GTP which acts at the N-protein to stimulate cAMP production, as does NaF. The fact that Gpp(NH)p and forskolin-stimulated adenylate cyclase activity does not change with age suggests that the N-protein and the catalytic unit do not change with age in this tissue.

No direct measurements of PTH-binding to renal membranes as a function of age have been made. However, several lines of evidence suggest there may be changes in PTH receptors with age. First, serum PTH levels increase with age in rats (5), and increased PTH levels have been shown to decrease renal

TABLE 3. Effect of age on adenylate cyclase activity of rat renal membranes[a]

Agonist	Adenylate cyclase activity (pmol cAMP/mg protein/min)	
	Young	Old
PTH (15 units/ml)	87 ± 2	49 ± 5[b]
Calcitonin (10 units/ml)	61 ± 1	75 ± 7
Gpp(NH)p (100 μM)	50 ± 7	51 ± 2
Forskolin (100 μM)	295 ± 24	315 ± 25

[a]Table entries are the mean ± SE of 3-4 replicates. Data from reference 6.
[b]Significantly different from young of same treatment group (P < 0.05, t-test).

receptor number (10). Secondly, if old rats are parathyroidectomized to remove endogenous PTH and reduce serum PTH levels, then PTH-sensitive adenylate cyclase activity is increased to the levels seen in young rats (6).

In contrast to PTH, calcitonin-stimulated adenylate cyclase shows no decrease with age (Table 3). This indicates that there is no change in the calcitonin receptor with age. This further suggests that in the kidney the N-protein and catalytic unit of adenylate cyclase do not change with age. The age-related changes in PTH and calcitonin-stimulated renal adenylate cyclase are summarized in Table 4.

TABLE 4. Summary of age-related changes in the adenylate cyclase complex of certain tissues

Tissue	Pathway	Receptor number	Receptor agonist affinity	N-protein	Catalytic unit
Human lymphocytes	beta-adrenergic	→[a]	↓	→	↓
Rat myocardium	beta-adrenergic	→	↓	↓	↓
Rat lung	beta-adrenergic	→	↓	—	↓
Rat kidney	parathyroid hormone	?↓	?↓	→	→
Rat kidney	calcitonin	→	→	→	→

[a]Arrows indicate increase (up), decrease (down), or no change (horizontal) in component with age. A dash indicates that changes were not studied. Question mark denotes indirect evidence.

COMPARISON OF AGE-RELATED CHANGES

From these studies, it is clear that there is no one defect that accounts for the age-related decrease in agonist-stimulated adenylate activity in all tissues (Table 4). The defects vary from tissue to tissue and some tissues contain more than one defect. In the beta-adrenergic pathways, there is no change in receptor numbers but there appears to be a decrease in the ability to form high affinity receptors and a decrease in catalytic unit activity in all tissues studied. In addition, the N-protein function decreases with age in the rat myocardium. On the other hand, in the rat kidney, N-protein and catalytic unit function do not change while receptor function appears to decrease.

The mechanisms responsible for these age-related changes in the components of the adenylate cyclase system remain to be elucidated. The decreased number of high affinity beta-adrenergic receptors may be related to the increases in catecholamine levels with age (13), but this remains to be demonstrated. In the kidney, alterations in the receptor appear closely tied to the age-related increase in serum PTH since parathyroid activity of old rats restores the renal adenylate cyclase response to that seen in young animals. The age-related changes in the N-protein and catalytic unit components could be due to a decreased number or decreased function of these components with age. These alterations remain to be explained at the molecular level.

The question also arises as to whether these age-related changes in adenylate cyclase activity account for the overall decline in hormone and drug action in these systems. Do the alterations in cAMP production result in alterations in cAMP-dependent protein kinase activity and the phosphorylation of specific proteins with age? In the heart, isoproterenol fully activated soluble protein kinase activity in all age groups. However, there was a decrease in the translocation of membrane-bound to soluble protein kinase activity with age (18). Likewise, PTH fully activated protein kinase in the kidney in all age groups (6). Membrane-bound protein kinase activity was not measured in this tissue. Further work is needed to determine if there are age-related changes in specific pools of protein kinase and in phosphorylation of specific proteins in these tissues.

CONCLUSION

There are significant changes in the adenylate cyclase complex of many tissues with age. These changes are not due to a single defect in the system. Rather, the defects may vary from tissue to tissue and may be multiple in nature. There are age-related changes described in the receptor, N-protein, and catalytic components of the adenylate cyclase system.

Alteration at the level of the receptor may reflect increases in the circulating levels of the agonist with age. The mechanisms responsible for alterations in the N-protein and catalytic unit activity remain to be elucidated. Further work is also needed to determine if the age-related changes in cAMP production result in age-related changes in cAMP-dependent protein kinase activity and the phosphorylation of specific proteins. However, the age-related changes in adenylate cyclase activity that have already been described may partially explain the decreased responsiveness of some target tissues to hormones and drugs.

ACKNOWLEDGMENTS

The authors gratefully acknowledge the excellent secretarial assistance of Yvonne Young. This research was supported by the Veterans Administration (HJA and PJS) and United States Public Health Services Grant AM 32158 (HJA).

REFERENCES

1. Abrass, I.B., and Scarpace, P.J. (1984): Clin. Res., 32:479a.
2. Abrass, I.B., and Scarpace, P.J. (1982): J. Clin. Endocrinol. Metab., 55:1026-1028.
3. Abrass, I.B., Davis, J.L., and Scarpace, P.J. (1982): J. Gerontol., 37:156-160.
4. Abrass, I.B., and Scarpace, P.J. (1981): J. Gerontol., 36:298-301.
5. Armbrecht, H.J., Forte, L.R., and Halloran, B.P. (1984): Am. J. Physiol., 246:E266-E270.
6. Armbrecht, H.J., Forte, L.R., Zenser, T.V., and Davis, B.B. (1984): Fed. Proc., 43(6):1580.
7. Armbrecht, H.J., Wongsurawat, N., Zenser, T.V., and Davis, B.B. (1982): Endocrinology, 111:1339-1344.
8. Feldman, R.D., Limbird, L.E., Nadeau, J., Robertson, D., and Wood, A.J.J. (1984): N. Engl. J. Med., 310:815-819.
9. Florini, J.R., and Regan, J.F. (1985): Rev. Biol. Res. Aging, 2:227-250.
10. Forte, L.R., Langelutting, S., Poelling, R.E., and Thomas, M.L. (1982): Am. J. Physiol., 242:E154-E163.
11. Gilman, A.G. (1984): Cell, 36:577-579.
12. Harden, T.K. (1983): Pharmacol. Rev., 35:5-32.
13. Krall, J.F., Connelly, M., Weisbart, R., and Tuck, M.L. (1981): J. Clin. Endocrinol. Metab., 52:863-867.
14. O'Connor, S.W., Scarpace, P.J., and Abrass, I.B. (1983): Mech. Ageing Dev., 21:357-363.
15. O'Connor, S.W., Scarpace, P.J., and Abrass, I.B. (1981): Mech. Ageing Dev., 16:91-95.
16. Scarpace, P.J., and Abrass, I.B. (1983): J. Gerontol., 38:143-147.

17. Scarpace, P.J., and Abrass, I.B. (1983): Gerontologist, 23:176.
18. Scarpace, P.J., and Abrass, I.B. (1985): Gerontologist, 25:448.
19. Seaman, K., and Daly, J.W. (1981): J. Biol. Chem., 256:9799-9801.
20. Sibley, D.R., and Lefkowitz, R.J. (1985): Nature, 317:124-129.
21. Tsai, K.-S., Heath, H., Kumar, R., and Riggs, B.L. (1984): J. Clin. Invest., 73:1668-1674.
22. Vestal, R.E., Wood, A.J.J., and Shand, D.G. (1979): Clin. Pharmacol. Ther., 26:181-185.

Subject Index

A

Adenylate cyclase system
  age-related changes in, 179–187
  components, 180–181
Adrenergic responsiveness, vascular
  in aging, 149–155
  homeostasis and, 154–155
Adrenergic system
  human lymphocytes and platelets and, 181–182
  rat heart and lung and, 182–184
Adverse drug interactions, in elderly, 141–146
  incidence and causative factors, 144–145
  theoretical basis, 141–144
Age changes
  in adenylate cyclase system, 179–187
    comparison of, 186
  in catalytic efficiency of MFOS enzymes, 165–167
  in immunological defense system, 131–138
  in liver MFOS components, 162–165
  in lung, 117–118
Age-related cognitive disturbances, pharmacological approaches, 74–85
Age-related memory problems, treatment, 71–85
Aged monkeys, *see* Monkeys, aged
Aging
  and blood pressure, 33–34
    alcohol consumption and, 29–44
  and host response to infectious disease, 107–112
  liver drug metabolism during, 159–175
Aging patients, compliance with antihypertensive therapy among, 6–9, 20–21; *see also* Elderly; Older populations
Alcohol consumption behaviors, and blood pressure, 34–41
Alcohol-induced dementias, 100–102
Alzheimer's disease
  future therapeutic strategies in, 65–66
  PNMT in, 56–60, 62–63
  loss of, mechanism for, 64–65
Animal preclinical research
  and human clinical, on age-related memory problems, 71–85
  on vascular adrenergic responsiveness in aging, 149–153

Antibiotic kinetics, in pneumonia, 121
Antibiotic treatment, of pneumonia in elderly, host defenses and, 115–126
Antibiotics, intracellular penetration of, in pneumonia, 125
Anticoagulants, in treatment of age-related cognitive disturbances
  clinical status, 77–78
  effects of, in aged monkeys, 78–79
Antihypertensive therapy
  approach of, 9–10
  benefits, 1–3
  compliance with, in older populations, 15–27
  of elderly, special considerations, 6–10

B

Blood pressure, *see also* Hypertension
  aging and, 33–34
  alcohol consumption behaviors and, 34–41
Blood pressure cuffs, experimental use of, 21–25
Brain, human, normal, PNMT in, 49–56
Brain function, PNMT neurons and, 60–61, 64

C

Calcitonin, parathyroid hormone and, system of, rat kidney and, 184–185
Catalytic efficiency, of MFOS enzymes, age changes in, 165–167
Central nervous system stimulants, in treatment of age-related cognitive disturbances
  clinical status, 79–80
  effects of, in aged monkeys, 80
Cerebral vasodilators, clinical status, in treatment of age-related cognitive disturbances, 77
Changes, age, *see* Age changes
Chemotherapy, response to, 111
Cholinomimetics, in treatment of age-related cognitive disturbances, clinical status and effects in aged monkeys, 83–85
Clinical manifestations, of infection, 109–110

189

Clinical status for treatment of age-related cognitive disturbances
  of anticoagulants (and rheologic agents), 77–78
  of central nervous system stimulants, 79–80
  of cerebral vasodilators, 77
  of cholinomimetics, 83–85
  of neuropeptides and other endogenous substances, 80–81
  of nootropics, 74–76
Cognitive disturbances, age-related, pharmacological approaches, 74–85
Cognitive functioning, 96
Complement factors, 136–137
Compliance, with antihypertensive therapy, 15–27
  among aging patients, 6–9, 20–21
  provider, patient and interaction problem in, 16–20
Confusion, 97–98
Cuffs, blood pressure, experimental use of, 21–25

D

Defense system, immunological, age and, 131–138
Defenses, host
  and antibiotic treatment of pneumonia in elderly, 115–126
  to infection, susceptibility and, 108–109
Delirium, 95
  drugs and, 98
  DSM III diagnostic criteria of, 97
Dementia(s), 96–97
  alcohol-induced, 100–102
  drug-induced, 98–100
  DSM III definition of, 95
Depression
  drugs and, 99–100
  DSM diagnostic criteria of, 98
Diagnosis, of pneumonia, see Pneumonia, diagnosis of
Disease
  Alzheimer's, see Alzheimer's disease
  infectious, host response to, aging and, 107–112
Disease states, underlying, pneumonia and, 117–118
Disturbances, cognitive, age-related, pharmacological approaches, 74–85
Drug-induced dementias, 98–100
Drug interactions, adverse, see Adverse drug interactions
Drug metabolism, liver, during aging, 159–175

E

Elderly, see also Age entries; Older population
  adverse drug interactions in, see Adverse drug interactions
  hypertension in, 1–11
  pneumonia in, antibiotic treatment of, host defenses and, 115–126
Endogenous substances, in treatment of age-related cognitive disturbances, clinical status of, 80–81
Enzymes, MFOS, age changes in catalytic efficiency of, 165–167
Etiology, of infections, 110–111
Experimental use, of blood pressure cuffs, 21–25

F

Future therapeutic strategies, in Alzheimer's disease, 65–66

G

Genetic expression of specific and nonspecific mediators, 131–138
Geriatric memory loss, probable causes, 73–74
Gram-negative pneumonia, treatment, 121–123
Gram-positive pneumonia, treatment, 123

H

Heart, and lung, rat, and adrenergic system, 182–184
Homeostasis, and vascular response, 154–155
Hormonal implications, pharmacological and, of age-related changes in adenylate cyclase system, 179–187
Hormone, parathyroid, and calcitonin, system of, rat kidney and, 184–185
Host defenses
  and antibiotic treatment of pneumonia in elderly, 115–126
  to infection, susceptibility and, 108–109
Host response, to infectious disease, aging and, 107–112
Human brain, normal, PNMT in, 49–56
Human lymphocytes, and platelets, adrenergic system and, 181–182
Human studies, of vascular adrenergic responsiveness in aging, 154
Hypertension, see also Antihypertensive therapy; Blood pressure
  in elderly, 1–11
  secondary, 5–6

SUBJECT INDEX

I

Immunological defense system, age and, 131–138
Immunoprophylaxis, response to, 111
Incidence, and causative factors, for drug interactions in elderly, 144–145
Infection(s)
 clinical manifestations, 109–110
 etiology, 110–111
 host defenses to, susceptibility and, 108–109
Infectious disease, host response to, aging and, 107–112
Interaction(s)
 adverse drug, see Adverse drug interactions
 physician/patient, problems in, and compliance with antihypertensive therapy, 19–20
Interleukins, 133–136
Intracellular penetration of antibiotics, in pneumonia, 125

K

Kidney, rat, and parathyroid hormone and calcitonin system, 184–185
Kinetics, antibiotic, in pneumonia, 121

L

Lipids, membrane, and MFOS activity, 168–171
Liver drug metabolism, during aging, 159–175
Liver MFOS components, age changes in, 162–165
Loss
 memory, geriatric, probable causes, 73–74
 of PNMT, in Alzheimer's disease, mechanism for, 64–65
Lung
 changes in, due to aging, 117–118
 rat heart and, and adrenergic system, 182–184
Lymphocytes, human, and platelets, adrenergic system and, 181–182

M

Mechanism, for loss of PNMT in Alzheimer's disease, 64–65
Mediators
 nonspecific, 136–137
 specific, 133–136
Membrane lipids, and MFOS activity, 168–171
Memory loss, geriatric, probable causes of, 73–74
Memory problems, age-related, treatment of, 71–85
Metabolism, drug, liver, during aging, 159–175
Mixed-function oxidase system (MFOS), 159
 activity
  membrane lipids and, 168–171
  nonhuman primate, 171–175
 components, liver, age changes in, 162–165
Mixed-function oxidase system enzymes, catalytic efficiency of, age changes in, 165–167
Monkeys, aged, and effects in treatment of age-related cognitive disturbances
 of anticoagulants, 78–79
 of central nervous system stimulants, 80
 of cholinomimetics, 83–85
 of neuropeptides, 82–83
 of nootropics, 76–77
Morbidity, and mortality, 107–108

N

Neurons, PNMT, and brain function, 60–61, 64
Neuropeptides, in treatment of age-related cognitive disturbances
 clinical status of, 80–81
 effects of, in aged monkeys, 82–83
Nonhuman primate MFOS activity, 171–175
Nonspecific mediators, 136–137
Nootropics, in treatment of age-related cognitive disturbances
 clinical status, 74–76
 effects of, in aged monkeys, 76–77
Normal human brain, PNMT in, 49–56
Normative Aging Study, 30–44
 blood pressure in, 33–34
  alcohol consumption behaviors and, 34–41

O

Older populations, compliance with antihypertensive therapy in, 15–27; see also Age entries; Elderly

P

Parathyroid hormone and calcitonin system, rat kidney and, 184–185
Patient(s)
 aging, compliance with antihypertensive therapy among, 20–21
 and compliance with antihypertensive therapy, 17–19
Penetration, intracellular, of antibiotics, in pneumonia, 125
Pharmacological approaches, for age-related cognitive disturbances, 74–85

Pharmacological implications, and hormonal, of age-related changes in adenylate cyclase system, 179–187
Phenylethanolamine *N*-methyltransferase (PNMT), 47
 in Alzheimer's disease, 56–60,62–63
 loss of, mechanism for, 64–65
 in normal human brain, 49–56
Phenylethanolamine *N*-methyltransferase neurons, and brain function, 60–61,64
Physicians, prescribing habits of, 19
Physiological considerations, in hypertension in elderly, 3–6
Platelets, human lymphocytes and, adrenergic system and, 181–182
Pneumonia, in elderly
 antibiotic kinetics in, 121
 antibiotic treatment of, host defenses and, 115–126
 diagnosis of, 118–120
  differential, 120
  factors affecting, 119–120
 gram-negative, treatment of, 121–123
 gram-positive, treatment of, 123
 intracellular penetration of antibiotics in, 125
 predisposition to, 117–118
 prevention, 120
 prognosis, 125–126
 treatment, 120–125
PNMT, *see* Phenylethanolamine *N*-methyltransferase
Preclinical research, animal
 and human clinical, on age-related memory problems, 71–85
 on vascular adrenergic responsiveness in aging, 149–153
Predisposition to pneumonia, 117–118
Prescribing habits, of physicians, 19
Prevention, of pneumonia, 120
Primate, nonhuman, MFOS activity in, 171–175
Problem(s)
 memory, age-related, treatment of, 71–85
 physician/patient interaction, and compliance with antihypertensive therapy, 19–20
Prognosis, in pneumonia, 125–126
Provider, and compliance with antihypertensive therapy, 19
Pseudohypertension, 4

R

Rat heart and lung, and adrenergic system, 182–184

Rat kidney, and parathyroid hormone and calcitonin system, 184–185
Response
 to chemotherapy, 111
 host, to infectious disease, aging and, 107–112
 to immunoprophylaxis, 111
 vascular adrenergic
  in aging, 149–155
  homeostasis and, 154–155
Rheologic agents, in treatment of age-related cognitive disturbances, clinical status of, 77–78
Rodent models, for liver drug metabolism during aging, 160–171

S

Secondary hypertension, 5–6
Specific mediators, 133–136
Stimulants, central nervous system, in treatment of age-related cognitive disturbances
 clinical status, 79–80
 effects of, in aged monkey, 80
Susceptibility, and host defenses to infection, 108–109

T

Theoretical basis, for adverse drug interactions, 141–144
Therapeutic strategies, future, in Alzheimer's disease, 65–66; *see also* Antihypertensive therapy; Treatment
Treatment
 of age-related memory problems, 71–85
 antibiotic, of pneumonia in elderly, host defenses and, 115–126
 for hypertension, *see* Antihypertensive therapy
 of pneumonia, 120–125

U

Underlying disease states, pneumonia and, 117–118

V

Vascular adrenergic responsiveness
 in aging, 149–155
 homeostasis and, 154–155